T3-BUV-615

Grand Rounds in Transplantation

Grand Rounds in Transplantation

J. Harold Helderman, M.D.
William H. Frist, M.D

The Vanderbilt Transplant Center

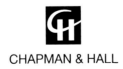

CHAPMAN & HALL

 An International Thomson Publishing Company

New York • Albany • Bonn • Boston • Cincinnati • Detriot • London • Madrid • Melbourne • Mexico City
Pacific Grove • Paris • San Francisco • Singapore • Tokyo • Toronto • Washington

Cover design: Trudi Gershenov

Copyright©1995
By Chapman & Hall
A division of International Thomson Publishing Inc.
IⓉP The ITP logo is a trademark under license

Printed in the United States of America

For more information, contact:

Chapman & Hall
One Penn Plaza
New York, NY 10119

International Thomson Publishing
Berkshire House 168-173
High Holborn
London WCIV 7AA
England

Thomas Nelson Australia
102 Dodds Street
South Melbourne, 3205
Victoria, Australia

Nelson Canada
1120 Birchmount Road
Scarborough, Ontario
Canada M1K 5G4

International Thomson Editores
Campos Eliseos 385, Piso 7
Col. Polanco
11560 Mexico D.F. Mexico

International Thomson Publishing Gmbh
Konigwinterer Strasse 418
53298 Bonn
Germany

International Thomson Publishing Asia
221 Henderson Road #05-10
Henderson Building
Singapore 0315

International Thomson Publishing—Japan
Hirakawacho-cho Kyowa Building, 3F
1-2-1 Hirakawacho-cho
Chiyoda-ku, 102 Tokyo
Japan

1 2 3 4 5 6 7 8 9 10 XXX 01 00 99 98 97 96 95

Library of Congress Catloging-in-Publication Data

Grand rounds in transplantation/[edited by] Harold J. Helderman, William H. Frist.
     p.   cm.
    Includes bibliographical references and index.
    ISBN 0-412-04271-1 (cloth) : $69.00
    1. Transplantation of organs, tissues, etc.--Complications--Case studies. I. Helderman, Harold J., 1945- . II. Frist, William H. [DNLM: 1. Transplantation--case studies. WO 660 G751 1995]
RD120.78.G73 1995
617.9'5--dc20
DNLM/DLC
for Library of Congress

94-22642
CIP

British Library Cataloguing in Publication Data available

Please send your order for this or any other Chapman & Hall book to **Chapman & Hall, 29 West 35th Street, New York, NY 10001, Attn: Customer Service Department.** You may also call our Order Department at 1-212-244-3336 or fax your purchase order to 1-800-248-4724.

For a complete listing of Chapman & Hall's titles, send your request to **Chapman & Hall, Dept. BC, One Penn Plaza, New York, NY 10119.**

To Phyllis and Karyn who have lovingly maintained the bedrock of our lives and families during many lonely hours in the operating theater, the hospital, on airplanes, and in foreign cities.

Contents

Preface

In 1991, the Nobel Committee recognized the importance of and the coming of age of transplantation when it gave its nod for the prize in medicine and physiology to Dr. Donnell Thomas and Dr. Joseph Murray. This joint award symbolized recognition of the practice of transplant by honoring two pioneers of the clinical wards and operating rooms rather than scientists of the growing, often arcane field of the immunobiology of transplantation, which had received earlier attention. Equally important symbolically was the joining of these two pioneers of different organs or tissues. Dr. Thomas was lauded for his work in bone marrow transplantation; whereas Dr. Murray was cited with his team for the initiation of clinical solid organ transplantation, in general, and kidney transplantation, in particular. The triumphs, the trials, the vicissitudes of the clinical practice of transplantation has importantly informed medicine and surgery in the late 20th century and will become, even more, a protean discipline for the 21st century. Our book has attempted to take cognizance of this expanding role for transplantation in the university hospital, the community hospital, and the medical school by bringing together a series of constructive case reports that span the issues of all transplantation as conducted at this time.

This book is a culmination of the vision of Vanderbilt University to bring the various transplant programs together under the umbrella of the Vanderbilt Transplant Center. All of the cases discussed in this book were encountered at Vanderbilt University Hospital, cared for by members of the Vanderbilt Transplant Center, and discussed by Center clinical scholars. Our goals are to be instructive and demonstrative. The cases seek to highlight classical problems encountered in the transplantation of the heart, the lung, the liver, the kidney, and the bone marrow cells. Many of the problems are typical of those encountered in a busy practice of transplantation. Some of the cases, while illustrating general points, do so with unusual presentations to heighten importance and interest in the general principle portrayed. All of the cases, taken together, are demonstrative of the collaborative efforts of the members of the transplant team, including our Center members involved in ethics, infectious disease, physiology, immunology, surgery, and medicine. They demonstrate both the unique problems of each organ but, more importantly, the common thread that binds the practice of transplantation together.

The first section deals with transplantation of the kidney. Three issues are discussed. First, the problem of recurrent disease after transplantation is dealt with by cases that illustrate frequent recurrence (hyperoxaluria) and a rarity (systemic lupus erythematosus). The reader is reminded that de novo glomerulonephritis is always a possibility with the illustration of a case of cryoglobulinemia. The ever-present problem of opportunistic infection in the immunocompromised transplant patient informs the remainder of the kidney transplant chapters with GU and GI histoplasmosis, a case of worm infestation, and a case of pulmonary cryptococcoses. Finally, neoplasia has always plagued organ transplantation, an observation highlighted by a case of severe Burkitt-like lymphoma.

The chapters of the heart transplant section deal with special problems of the transplant of that organ. A chapter on the technique to transplant a heart into a child previously repaired for congenital heart disease is such. Two chapters dealing with the diagnosis of acute and chronic rejection by newer modalities are followed by a chapter on the treatment of a major complication of heart transplant, the vasculopathy culminating in atherosclerosis. The last chapter illustrates the breadth of concern in this grand round series, a chapter dealing with the ethical issues raised by heart transplantation into an expanding population, in this case the elderly.

Lung transplantation is represented by a case of the most important complication, acute bronchiolitis obliterans. This problem of lung transplant has been felt to be the manner in which lung vessels react to acute rejection. A second patient is discussed for which photopheresis was employed to treat chronic rejection of the lung.

Liver transplantation deals especially with transplantation for viral hepatitis which may reoccur after engraftment. Chapter 16 and 17 deals with this very important issue with cases of hepatitis C and hepatitis B. Multiple postengraftment complications related to surgery and its medical complications are addressed with cases detailing a variceal hemorrhage and hypovitaminosis due to reduction or absence of bile flow. The last chapter in this section deals with a bioartifical liver as an option for the treatment of liver failure as a bridge to transplantation.

The last section of the book deals with bone marrow transplantation. Chapter 21 addresses the very important issue of the appropriate stem cell source for reconstitution of patients for the most effective bone marrow transplant engraftment. Two devastating complications are discussed, a case of graft-versus-host disease and a case of veno-occlusive disease of the liver after bone marrow transplantation. Finally, infections are among the most important issues dealt with in the bone marrow transplant arena and are discussed with a case of nocardia and a case of adenovirus.

This book deals with the wide range of problems encountered in a vigorous transplant practice using a case-report-driven format. This format allows for single problems to be underscored in the practice of transplant medicine. The distinctive features of this book include issues that encompass a wide experience in transplantation including heart, lung, kidney, liver, and bone marrow transplantation. Equally unique is the inclusion of issues that involve the ethics of transplantation, the psychology of transplantation, and the practice of infectious disease as it applies to transplantation coupled to the usual concerns of immunobiology, immunosuppression, and the management and diagnosis of rejection.

These case-reports-driven lessons each make important points of the practice of transplantation. It has been our pleasure to put together these cases, co-author several of them, and make them available to the interested reader in this era of expanding transplantation presence.

1

Primary Hyperoxaluria

*Bryan Becker, Christina Ynares,
and J. Harold Helderman*

CASE HISTORY

A 27-year-old male with a history of primary hyperoxaluria presented for his second living-related donor renal transplantation.

Twelve years prior to admission, the patient developed symptoms of an upper respiratory tract infection. One month later, he presented to his physician in Florida complaining of anorexia, pruritus, neuromuscular instability, and malaise. Clinical and laboratory evaluation revealed uremia as the cause of his symptoms. Serum chemistries at that time were remarkable for blood urea nitrogen = 234 mg/dl and serum creatinine = 26 mg/dl.

The patient underwent thorough evaluation for the etiology of his renal failure. Serologic tests including antinuclear antibody and hepatitis B surface antigen were negative. Serum C3 level = 16 U/ml was slightly depressed, whereas an antistreptolysin titer = 250 Todd units was mildly elevated and anti-DNA was positive. The patient then underwent a DTPA renal scan which demonstrated absent flow and no function in both kidneys. A retrograde pyelogram displayed a staghorn calculus in the right renal pelvis and nephrocalcinosis involving the left kidney. The etiology of his renal disease was presumed chronic glomerulonephritis and idiopathic nephrocalcinosis, and the patient was initiated on hemodialysis. A right Cimino fistula was placed and the patient continued hemodialysis near his home in Florida. The patient was subsequently referred to our institution for possible living-related donor renal transplantation.

In July 1979, he underwent bilateral nephrectomy and renal transplantation (donated by his father) without complications. Pathologic examination of the native kidneys revealed numerous changes. These included tubular atrophy, birefringent crystals, chronic inflammation in the interstitium, and massive calcium oxalate deposits. Renal calculi removed at time of transplantation were analyzed and shown to be 100% calcium oxalate. The serum creatinine fell rapidly postoperatively to 2.2 mg/dl and the patient maintained good urine output without requiring dialysis. Prior to discharge, a plasma oxalate level was obtained, 4.65 μg/ml (nl 1–2.4), as was a 24-h urine collection for oxalate, 148 mg/ 24 h (nl 0–45).

The patient experienced an episode of acute rejection in July 1980 treated successfully with high-dose intravenous corticosteroids. In January 1981, he again experienced an episode of acute rejection. Renal biopsy at that time, however, also displayed recurrent calcium oxalate deposits. A follow-up 24-h urine collection for oxalate 2 months later continued to demonstrate significant oxaluria, 141 mg/24 h.

The patient's graft never achieved "normal" function. His serum creatinine hovered between 2.5 and 3.0 mg/dl. By February 1982, the patient's renal function had further deteriorated. His serum creatinine had gradually increased to 4.2 mg/dl. A renogram showed a marked decrease in function of the transplant kidney. The patient then underwent open renal biopsy. Pathologic findings visualized in the biopsy specimen included widening of the lamina rara interna and fusion of epithelial cell foot processes. There was also an increase in mesangial matrix and further calcium oxalate deposition. These were consistent with oxalate nephropathy and transplant glomerulopathy. The patient was discharged from the hospital and returned to hemodialysis soon thereafter. His medications at that time included prednisone, azathioprine, cimetidine, ferrous sulfate, methylene blue, and pyridoxine.

He underwent cadaveric renal transplantation in December 1982. This graft provided excellent function for nearly 4 years before the patient again developed progressive renal insufficiency. Renal biopsy performed in early 1987 demonstrated chronic rejection with rare oxalate crystals, and the patient returned to hemodialysis in May 1987.

He was maintained on high-dose pyridoxine and methylene blue after both transplants as therapy for his oxalosis. A transplant nephrectomy of his first graft was performed in 1988 secondary to fever, graft pain, and tenderness over the kidney. Pathology of this kidney revealed extensive crystalline oxalate deposition, nephrocalcinosis, and rejection.

The patient continued on hemodialysis and pursued evaluation for dual hepatic–renal transplantation. A second living-related donor kidney transplant was planned. In an effort to normalize oxalate metabolism and prevent rapid recurrence of oxalosis in this new renal transplant, the patient underwent intraperitoneal implantation of heterologous hepatocytes in early July 1990. Further transplantation workup was hampered by persistently elevated panel reactive antibodies (PRA). In order to ameliorate this immunologic obstacle he received immunoadsorption therapy per protocol as well as pretransplant administration of antithymocyte serum in preparation for this living-related renal transplant from a 3 antigen match sibling in mid-July 1990.

The patient's medications included prednisone 5 mg twice daily, cyclosporine A 150 mg twice daily, cimetidine 300 mg at night, ferrous sulfate 325 mg three times daily, a daily vitamin supplement, calcitriol 0.25 μg daily, and erythropoietin 3000 units three times weekly after dialysis.

On physical examination, the patient was a thin emaciated male in no acute distress. Vital signs were T = 36.8°C, BP = 112/72 mm Hg, HR = 82/min, RR = 20/min. The remainder of the examination was remarkable for a healed midline surgical incision as well as healed right and left lower quadrant transverse incisions and a well-healed right lower quadrant paramedian incision. Head and neck examination was unremarkable. Chest auscultation revealed clear lung fields and a soft II/VI systolic murmur along the left sternal border. His abdomen was flat and nontender with normoactive bowel sounds. A right forearm Goretex shunt was also nontender and demonstrated a palpable thrill and audible bruit. There were femoral bruits bilaterally and moderately decreased posterior tibial and dorsalis pedis pulses bilaterally. The only other remarkable finding was the patient's upper extremity tremor. Pertinent laboratory studies and radiographs are shown in Table 1-1.

After vigorous daily preoperative hemodialysis and the aforementioned experimental therapies, the patient underwent living-related kidney transplantation. The donor kidney had two small arteries, each approximately 2.5 mm in diameter. After successful vascular anastamoses, the transplanted kidney began to perfuse and produce urine. Almost immediately postoperatively however, urine production precipitously declined and the patient became anuric. A renogram performed on postoperative day 1 showed no blood flow to the kidney. In spite of adequate volume replacement, anuria persisted and he underwent hemofiltration.

Table 1-1. Laboratory Data on Admission

Serum Na	134 mEq/l
Serum K	3.8 mEq/l
Serum Cl	94 mEq/l
Serum HCO_3	29 mEq/l
Serum BUN	62 mg/dl
Serum Cr	6.5 mg/dl
WBC	4000/mm^3
Hgb	7.2 mg/dl
Hct	22%
Platelet	229,000/mm^3
SGOT	34 U/L
Alk Phos	198 U/L
T Bili	0.7 mg/dl
Serum Ca	8.4 mEq/l
Serum PO_4	5.8 mEq/l
Albumin	3.1 mg/dl
ECG	Sinus rhythm, rate 90
CXR	Mild cardiomegaly, no edema

Grave concern arose regarding the possibility of hyperacute rejection. On postoperative day 2, the patient returned to the operating room for transplant nephrectomy. At the time of surgery the kidney appeared to have no arterial flow. The allograft was then removed without complications. Pathologic examination of the kidney demonstrated tubular necrosis without inflammation and small arterial thrombi. No features of hyperacute rejection were present. The patient recovered thereafter and returned to hemodialysis.

Over the ensuing $1\frac{1}{2}$ he sustained multiple episodes of digital gangrene related to vascular insufficiency. He also developed a severely disabling osteodystrophy. A bone marrow biopsy in early 1992 demonstrated diffuse oxalate deposition, again consistent with his underlying disease. He underwent several additional vascular access procedures secondary to clotting but gradually succumbed to poor nutrition, end-stage renal disease, and the complications of his underlying disease. He died in 1992, almost 13 years after his initial presentation.

DISCUSSION

The Disease

The patient presented herein suffered from a rare inborn error of metabolism, primary hyperoxaluria type 1 (PH1). First described by Lepoutre in 1925, this autosomal recessive disease stems from a functional deficiency of the enzyme, alanine glyoxylate aminotransferase (AGT: EC 2.6.1.44) in hepatic peroxisomes. The lack of functional enzyme results in continued overabundant synthesis and excretion of oxalic acid as well as glyoxylate and glycolic acid (see Fig. 1-1). Over time, this leads to systemic calcium oxalate deposition. The sequelae of this condition are many and include recurrent nephrolithiasis, nephrocalcinosis, and

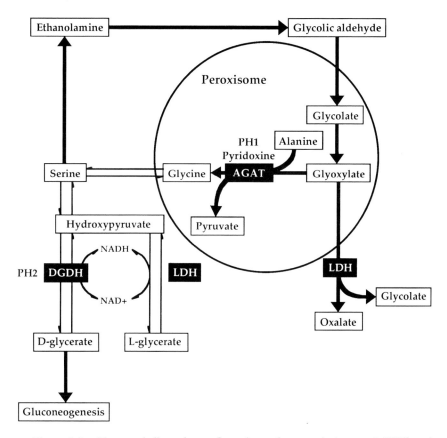

Figure 1-1. The metabolic pathways for primary hyperoxaluria type 1 (PH1) and primary hyperoxaluria type 2 (PH2). In PH1, hepatic peroxisomes are deficient in functional alanine:glyoxylate aminotransferase (AGT). In PH2, there is deficient extraperoxisomal D-glyceric acid dehydrogenase. AGT = alanine:glyoxylate aminotransferase; DGDH = D-glyceric acid dehydrogenase; LDH = lactate dehydrogenase; NADH = reduced nicotinamide adenine nucleotide; NAD+ = nicotinamide adenine dinucleotide. (Used with permission from Small KW, Scheinman J, Klintworth GK. A clinicopathological study of ocular involvement in primary hyperoxaluria type I. *Br J Ophthamol* 1992 76:54–57.)

progressive renal failure (see Table 1-2). This disease obviously carries a high morbidity as evidenced by the difficult course of the aforementioned patient. Primary hyperoxaluria, however, is doubly disheartening secondary to its tremendous mortality. More than 50% of patients with PH1 are dead by age 13 if left untreated. Greater than 55% of patients with PH1 die by the age of 20 and only 15% of patients are still alive at the age of 35.

Other forms of genetic hyperoxaluria exist. An in-depth discussion of these entities is beyond the scope of this chapter. For more information the reader is referred to excellent reviews by Smith and Hillman.

Briefly however, type 2 primary hyperoxaluria is also an autosomal recessive disorder. Here, a deficiency of glyoxylate reductase [D-glycerate dehydrogenase (EC 1.1.1.29)] is present, resulting in many findings similar to PH1, including renal failure. The major difference between this entity and PH1 is the enzymatic defect and its cellular distribution. A specific deficiency in leukocyte D-glyceric dehydrogenase has been uncovered in a small number of patients. This results in excessive urinary excretion of oxalic acid and L-glyceric acid but not glycolic acid nor glyoxylate.

Isolated hyperabsorption of oxalate without any frank intestinal disease is the underlying cause for type 3 primary hyperoxaluria. Experience with this disease entity is limited, but it has not been associated with any other organic aciduria to date. Finally, mention should be made of secondary hyperoxaluria. This may arise in the setting of inflammatory bowel disease, after jejunoileal bypass, or simply upon ingestion of large amounts of oxalate or oxalate precursors. These latter scenarios rarely result in end-stage renal disease.

As noted, patients with PH1 suffer not only from an excessive pro-

Table 1-2. Systemic Manifestations of Primary Hyperoxaluria

Nephrolithiasis
Nephrocalcinosis
Renal insufficiency
Uremia
Conduction system abnormalities (A-V block)
Dilated cardiomyopathy
Arthritis
Osteopathy
Vascular insufficiency
Retinopathy
Neuropathy

duction of oxalate but also an inability to excrete this tremendous oxalate burden with renal deposition of oxalate (see Fig. 1-2). Calcium oxalate, thus, deposits at both intrarenal and extrarenal sites. When calcium oxalate involves the kidney, it manifests itself as recurrent nephrolithiasis and/or nephrocalcinosis. The aforementioned patient suffered from both of these complications and progressed to end-stage renal failure as do most patients with PH1.

Extrarenal deposition of calcium oxalate is one of the hallmarks of primary hyperoxaluria. When this transpires in a patient's course, it is termed *oxalosis*. Extensive crystalline deposits of calcium oxalate can involve many different organ systems. Classically, however, calcium oxalate attacks the musculoskeletal system, the vasculature, and the heart. It can precipitate within joints, resulting in an acute gout-like arthritis. Chronic bony changes develop when calcium oxalate deposits along bony metaphyses within tubular bones, giving rise to oxalate osteopathy. Calcium oxalate crystals can also accumulate in large vessels and lead to progressive vascular insufficiency. Patients usually develop vascular bruits or may even suffer the devastating consequences of limb or digital infarction as our patient demonstrated. Rarely, they will evolve an acute livedo reticularis mimicking cholesterol embolization. Calcium oxalate also deposits within the heart and, specifically, within its conduction system. Frequently, cardiovascular involvement contributes to the early mortality in individuals with PH1. Patients can develop a diffuse dilated cardiomyopathy, but, more often, they display a variety of dysrhythmias and often suffer from symptomatic atrioventricular block.

PH1 as a disease displays tremendous heterogeneity at both the clinical and molecular levels. Clinically, this disease manifests significant variability in the age of onset (<1 year to >55 years), age at death (<1 year to >65 years), and symptomatology. The proportional effects of nephrocalcinosis, nephrolithiasis, and systemic oxalosis differ markedly among patients. The degrees of hyperoxaluria and hyperglycolic aciduria also vary greatly among individuals. Disease progression displays similar heterogeneity, with some patients appearing relatively unaffected for years, whereas others succumb to PH1 readily. The lone caveat related to progression is the inevitable development of end-stage renal disease soon after the glomerular filtration rate (GFR) falls below 40 ml/min.

The protean nature of PH1 extends to the molecular level and its enzymatic expression. The putative gene harboring human AGT is located on chromosome 2q36-q37. Investigations by Danpure [1] have demonstrated extensive enzyme heterogeneity in this disorder. Liver samples were taken from 58 patients afflicted with PH1 and analyzed

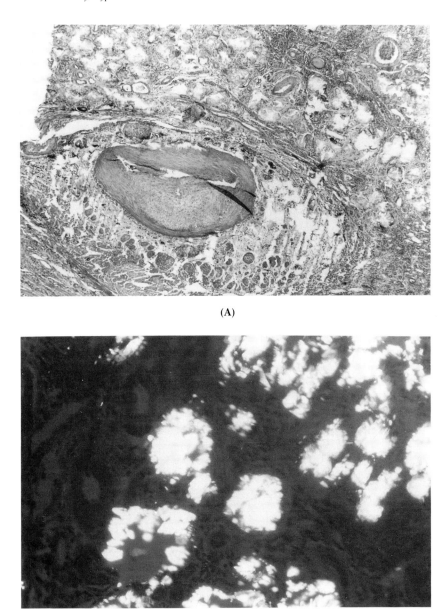

(A)

(B)

Figure 1-2. (*A*) Kidney tissue removed at the time of nephrectomy (magnification ×150). (*B*) The same specimen visualized under polarized microscopy (magnification ×150) demonstrating the marked burden of oxalate crystals throughout the kidney.

for peroxisomal alanine:glyoxylate aminotransferase (AGT) activity. Approximately 60% of PH1 patients had zero AGT catalytic activity, whereas the remaining 40% of patients displayed 3–48% of the mean normal enzymatic catalytic activity. The hepatic samples were also examined for the presence of cross-reacting material/immunoreactive AGT protein (CRM). All patients with AGT expressed CRM as well; but, interestingly, several patients without AGT activity also expressed CRM. More importantly, Danpure further evaluated the subcellular location of AGT and CRM in these patients. The majority of patients expressing both AGT activity and CRM had hepatic AGT localized to the wrong intracellular compartment, that is, mitochondria. Thus, Danpure has suggested that a unique trafficking defect may be responsible for some of the variability seen in PH1.

Diagnosis and Therapy

With such a course, early diagnosis of PH1 is imperative to plan therapeutic strategies. The majority of patients will present with symptoms of nephrolithiasis either as asymptomatic hematuria or as typical renal colic. Other individuals such as the aforementioned patient can present with uremia and no previous history of clinical stone disease. Less commonly, patients will come to medical attention manifesting renal failure and cystic bony lesions. In these instances, bone biopsy aids in the diagnosis of oxalosis.

Various examination, laboratory, and radiographic abnormalities may be helpful in documenting PH1. No singular finding, however, is pathognomonic for the disease. As noted above, skeletal x-rays in affected patients can reveal changes consistent with oxalate osteopathy. Individuals can suffer retinal infarcts demonstrable on funduscopic examination or they can display signs of peripheral vascular disease. Urinary oxalate crystals are usually identifiable in patients with PH1, but their presence is highly nonspecific. Similarly, the finding of nephrocalcinosis on renal ultrasound in a patient with idiopathic renal failure heightens the suspicion for PH1 but demands further evaluation.

Traditionally, the diagnosis of PH1 has rested upon the presence of elevated urinary oxalate (>45 mg/day in adults) and glycolate in the absence of other attributable causes, for example, primary bowel disease or pyridoxine deficiency. Notably, up to one-third of PH1 patients will have normal urinary glycolate levels. Because obvious difficulties exist when trying to obtain timed urine collections in infants and children, the simpler measure, a urinary oxalate/creatinine ratio, has been advocated, at least as a diagnostic guideline. Values >0.3 mg in infants,

>0.1 mg in children ages 1–5 years, and >0.05 mg in children over 5 years are strongly suggestive of PH1 and require further investigation. The actual utility of liver biopsy and direct hepatic determination of AGT levels is limited at present but may be necessarily justified to make an enzyme-deficiency diagnosis.

Once PH1 is identified, several general measures can be undertaken to stem its complications. Initial therapy consists primarily of treatment to prevent stone formation. Sufficient fluid intake is important as is a diet low in oxalate, calcium, and only the minimum requirements for vitamins C and D. Dietary modifications will obviously have to be made to accommodate growing children with this disorder. Prompt treatment of urinary tract infections is essential as well.

Potentially useful medications include pyridoxine (B_6), orthophosphate, magnesium, and thiazide diuretics. Pyridoxine treatment provides the necessary cofactor for all aminotransferases, pyridoxal phosphate (see Fig. 1-1). Hence, its utility is specific for PH1. A small minority of patients will respond marvelously to physiologic doses of pyridoxine (2–10 mg/day). These patients are pyridoxine-sensitive and may need no additional therapy. A far larger number of PH1 patients, however, will require large doses of pyridoxine (200–400 mg/day) to decrease measured oxalate excretion. Neutral orthophosphate (0.5–1.5 g/day) and magnesium gluconate (1 g/day) were historically advocated as combination medications to inhibit crystallization. Their efficacy was established by Smith and Williams and subsequent authors who have corraborated their results. The mechanisms by which these medications alter stone formation are still unclear. Orthophosphate administration appears to act by two different modes. First, it decreases calcium absorption and thereby decreases urinary calcium. Second, it increases urinary excretion of pyrophosphate which inhibits calcium oxalate crystal growth. Magnesium also affects calcium oxalate solubility, thus, diminishing crystal deposition.

In the setting of proven hypercalciuria, thiazide diuretics can be added to this regimen to reduce the urinary calcium concentration. Some authors have also suggested citrate as adjunctive therapy to further alter crystal formation [9]. This has the potential, however, to aggravate preexisting hypocalcemia. As such, its use should be reserved for patients with significant acidosis. Finally, monitoring of serum calcium, phosphate, alkaline phosphatase, and urine calcium is warranted during treatment with any of these agents to identify the insidious evolution of hyperparathyroidism.

Obviously, the aforementioned medications should continue even as renal failure develops. Persistent close follow-up becomes imperative to avoid hyperphosphatemia, and, if identified, orthophosphate should be discontinued immediately. All these measures will, nonetheless, decrease in effectiveness as GFR declines to ≤ 20 ml/min and renal failure begins to intervene. Elegant radioisotope analyses and serial measurements of plasma oxalate have demonstrated expansion of the metabolic oxalate pool and accelerated oxalate deposition as renal failure ensues. This results in the systemic oxalosis so frequently seen in end-stage patients with PH1 and heralds mortality if left unchecked. For these reasons, many authors have suggested that plans for definitive treatment should be solidified and undertaken as the patient's GFR falls to ≤ 20 ml/min.

Aggressive dialysis, though obviously essential for individuals with renal failure, is only of minimal benefit in reducing the oxalate burden in patients with systemic oxalosis. Classic studies performed by Watts et al. [2] in the mid-1980s evaluated oxalate dynamics and removal rates with both peritoneal dialysis and hemodialysis. They concluded that standard hemodialysis was more efficient than peritoneal dialysis at reducing serum oxalate concentrations. Nevertheless, neither mode of dialysis could match the rapid rate of tissue oxalate accretion seen in patients with primary hyperoxaluria. Other investigators have examined the capacity for high-flux hemodialysis to remove oxalate in patients end stage renal disease. Highly permeable polyacrylonitrile (AN-69) membranes provided more efficient oxalate clearance than standard cuprophane membranes; however, ultimately, there were no significant differences in plasma oxalate concentrations nor oxalate metabolic pool sizes in patients undergoing either form of dialysis. Further studies are thus needed to analyze whether intensive dialysis regimens, hemofiltration, or high-flux hemodialysis are truly of demonstrable benefit in this setting.

Transplantation

At present, the most efficacious treatment for pyridoxine-resistant PH1 as well as the other primary hyperoxalurias is transplantation. Renal transplantation alone in PH1 has met with, at best, limited success. Data reported by Broyer et al. [3] examined renal transplantation in a population of 221 patients with PH1. Ninety-eight of these patients received kidney transplants, of which 79 were from cadaveric donors. Only 45% of these grafts remained functional at 6 months and nearly 85% had failed by 36 months. Even the living-related (LRD) transplants demonstrated decreased graft survival. Almost 40% of these transplants had failed by 1 year and only 23% were functioning at 36 months.

The most common reason for graft failure aside from rejection was the rapid recurrence of nephrocalcinosis in the transplant kidney. This bore out the conclusion that graft survival was dependent, at least, in part, on the patient's preexisting oxalate load. A large oxalate burden resulted in a poorer prognosis for graft survival. As such, transplant protocols have been subsequently designed to provide intensive pre-transplant dialysis to remove as much oxalate as possible. Additionally, early posttransplant diuresis has been aggressively pursued to dilute the oxalate being mobilized and presented to the new kidney. Any and all other potentially helpful therapies, for example, pyridoxine, ortho-phosphate, and even posttransplant dialysis, have been utilized to con-fer the greatest possible advantage to graft survival.

With these objectives in mind, several groups have demonstrated ad-equate results with regard to short-term graft survival. Scheinman et al. [4] achieved graft survival and good renal function in 7/10 LRD transplant recipients up to 7 years after transplantation. Watts et al. [5, 6] employed similar measures but only 2/6 renal transplant recipients had functioning grafts at 18 months after transplantation. A third pa-tient suffered cyclosporine toxicity as the etiology of graft failure, whereas the remaining three individuals all developed recurrent renal oxalate deposition. Nevertheless, these results were encouraging as they vali-dated several factors favoring successful renal transplantation including early transplantation, high-volume urine flow, and vigorous hemodi-alysis preoperatively and postoperatively, if necessary, to diminish the oxalate metabolic pool. Watts et al. [5, 6] also concluded that LRD grafts were not necessarily better than cadaveric grafts for transplantation, thus freeing PH1 patients from the stringent LRD criterion.

Liver transplantation offers the salient advantage of providing the normal enzyme, AGT, in its appropriate milieu [10, 11]. The first liver transplant for PH1 was performed in 1985 by Watts. This individual underwent combined hepatic and renal transplantation. Though the patient died postoperatively, there was clear evidence of diminished rates of oxalate production and shrinkage of the metabolic oxalate pool.

Subsequent to this biochemical success orthotopic liver transplanta-tion usually with associated renal transplantation has been advocated a therapy for primary hyperoxaluria. In the largest series published to date, nine patients have been treated with this combination procedure. Four of the nine patients survived (22–39 months follow-up) with asymptomatic resolution of their oxalosis. One sustained hyperacute re-jection, leading to loss of the renal transplant. The remaining four in-dividuals died 0–14 months after transplant. Notably, despite normalization of oxalate production, each survivor still displayed elevated levels of urinary oxalate excretion.

To minimize the potential threat of graft failure posed by the systemic oxalate burden, alternative transplantation strategies have been proposed. A two-stage procedure involving sequential hepatic then renal transplantation has been performed. Hepatic transplantation presumptively should decrease excess oxalate synthesis and partially diminish the metabolic oxalate pool prior to renal transplantation. This approach has met with clinical success. Liver transplantation alone has been attempted as well in one instance with positive results, including resolution of renal oxalate deposition. Heterotopic auxiliary liver transplantation and hepatocyte implantation have been proposed and attempted as in this patient's history. Results have been variable at best. Theoretical arguments have been postulated for their lack of success. These include competition from the patient's own liver which functions normally aside from AGT deficiency and the lengthy course glyoxylate must traverse from patient hepatocyte to donor hepatocyte without undergoing conversion to oxalate.

Certainly, in providing the missing enzyme, liver transplantation is curative therapy for PH1. Various authors have recommended that hepatic transplantation proceed once the patient's GFR declines to approximately 20 ml/min. Systemic oxalosis is reversible in this setting and should not discourage transplantation. A caveat applies here, however, as Watts has suggested advanced osteodystrophy, oxalate vasculopathy, and diffuse subcutaneous calcinosis serve as relative contraindications to transplantation. Interestingly, resolution of oxalate osteopathy in a patient who underwent combined liver–kidney transplantation has recently been reported. Thus, the first entity in this list in time may not even be considered a relative contraindication to combined organ transplantation. As further experience is gained, it appears that hepatic transplantation will become the indicated standard therapy for PH1 as renal function deteriorates. At present, however, renal transplantation still provides good results and, thus, remains the preferred first choice by many physicians.

SUMMARY

Primary hyperoxaluria is an autosomal recessive disorder typified by excessive urinary excretion of glyoxylic and glycolic acids. It results from a deficiency of alanine:glyoxylate aminotransferase, an enzyme localized to hepatic peroxisomes. The manifestations of primary hyperoxaluria range from nephrolithiasis and nephrocalcinosis to oxalate vasculopathy, retinopathy, osteopathy, and even cardiac involvement. The prognosis for this disease is poor if left untreated. Initial modes of therapy consist of measures to delay stone formation and the progression of renal failure. Subsequent organ transplantation (hepatic or hepatic–renal) can be of great benefit and, even, curative.

REFERENCES

1. Danpure CJ. Molecular and clinical heterogeneity in primary hyperoxaluria type 1. *Am J Kidney Dis* 1991;17:366–369.
2. Watts RWE, Veall N, Purkiss P. Oxalate dynamics and removal rates during haemodialysis and peritoneal dialysis in patients with primary hyperoxaluria and renal failure. *Clin Sci* 1984;66:591–597.
3. Broyer M, Brunner FP, Brynger H et al. Kidney transplantation in primary oxalosis: Data from the EDTA Registry. *Nephrol Dial Transplant* 1990;5:332–336.
4. Scheinman JL. Therapy for primary hyperoxaluria. *Kidney Int* 1991;40:389–399.
5. Watts RWE, Morgan SH, Danpure CJ et al. Combined hepatic and renal transplantation in primary hyperoxaluria type 1: Clinical report of nine cases. *Am J Med* 1991;90:179–188.
6. Watts RWE, Danpure CJ, DePauw L et al. Combined liver–kidney and isolated liver transplantations for primary hyperoxaluria type 1: The European experience. *Nephrol Dial Transplant* 1991;6:502–511.
7. Hillman RE. Primary hyperoxalurias. In: Scriver CR, Beaudet AL, Sly WS, Valle D eds. *The Metabolic Basis of Inherited Disease*. New York: McGraw Hill, 1989:933–944.
8. Williams HE, Smith LH. L-Glyceric aciduria: a new genetic variant of primary hyperoxaluria. *N Engl J Med* 1968;278:233–239.
9. Watts RWE. Treatment of renal failure in the primary hyperoxalurias. *Nephron* 1990;56:1–5.
10. Cochat P, Faure JL, Divry P et al. Liver transplantation in primary hyperoxaluria type 1. *Lancet* 1989;1:1142–1143.
11. Toussaint C, DePauw L, Vienne A et al. Radiological and histological improvement of oxalate osteopathy after combined liver-kidney transplantation in primary hyperoxaluria type 1. *Am J Kidney Dis* 1993;21:54–63.

2

Renal Allograft Dysfunction More Than 10 Years After Transplant in a Lupus Patient

Mahendra V. Govani, Agnes Fogo, and Christina Ynares

CASE PRESENTATION

History

A 50-year-old Caucasian man was admitted on 2 November 1993 for transplant renal biopsy because of fluid retention and increasing serum creatinine. He had a 2A, 2B matched living-related kidney transplant from his brother in 1983 for end-stage renal disease (ESRD) secondary to systemic lupus erythematosus (SLE).

Seventeen years before admission, he was admitted for bilateral pleural effusions, proteinuria, hematuria, and impaired renal function. Diagnosis of SLE was made on the basis of clinical findings, positive lupus serology, and characteristic findings on renal biopsy. The biopsy showed WHO class IV lupus nephritis characterized by diffuse segmental proliferative glomerulonephritis with discontinuous capillary loop staining for IgG, IgM, C3, and C4 by immunofluorescence. Electron microscopy showed abundant subendothelial and mesangial dense deposits with occasional subepithelial deposits and numerous reticular aggregates in endothelial cell cytoplasm. He was started on high doses of oral glucocorticoids, and azathioprine was added after a month. His proteinuria improved significantly and serum creatinine stabilized around 2 mg/dl. He developed diabetes mellitus approximately 3 months after he was started on glucocorticoids, treated with diet restriction and insulin. In October 1980, he developed significant proximal myopathy related to the high dose of glucocorticoids, therefore, the dose of prednisone was reduced. His azathioprine was also stopped at the time. His renal function gradually deteriorated and he was started on hemodialysis in March 1983. In July 1983, he had a living-related kidney transplant from his brother. During transplant surgery, a splenic artery aneurysm (approximately 1.5 cm in diameter) was found and the splenic artery was ligated. He also had a proximal gastric vagotomy at the time because of his long-standing history of peptic ulcer disease.

In March 1977, pulmonary tuberculosis was diagnosed and he was treated with antituberculous therapy. In February 1978, he had an appendectomy for acute appendicitis. A Clark's level II melanoma was removed from his left forearm in 1978. In August 1985, a basal cell carcinoma was excised from the left side of his nose. In September 1985, an exploratory laparotomy performed for abdominal pains revealed adhesions from previous surgery. In October 1986, he was admitted with an acute inferior wall myocardial infarction. In October 1987, he had a right orchiectomy for chronic suppurative epididymoorchitis. In January 1993, he was admitted with unstable angina. Cardiac catheterization showed moderate two vessel disease and mild hypokinesia of the inferior wall; however, the overall left ventricular function was normal. His angina was controlled with medications.

For 10 years following transplantation, his renal function remained stable with serum creatinine less than 1.2 mg/dl and no proteinuria on urinanalysis. He did not have any episode of rejection or flare-up of SLE. He had several episodes of urinary tract infections which responded promptly to antibiotics.

Nine weeks before admission, at his last hospital visit, he was asymptomatic; his physical examination was unremarkable and his laboratory values were unchanged from the previous visit.

Two weeks before admission, he noticed diminished urine output and swelling of the legs. He also complained of generalized weakness, tiredness, and vague headaches. There was no history of dysuria, abdominal pains, nausea, vomiting, diarrhea, arthritis, arthralgia, skin rash, cough, chest pain, or dyspnea.

His medications on admission were Imuran 50 mg QD, prednisone 5 mg BID, Procardia, Corgard, Bactrim DS, and NPH insulin QAM. He had smoked 1–2 packs of cigarettes per day all his adult life without any intention of stopping smoking. He was noncompliant with his follow-up appointments and probably medications. There was no family history of SLE, diabetes mellitus, hypertension, or renal disease.

Physical Examination

Vitals: pulse 64/min and regular, BP 168/77 mm Hg, temperature 98.5°F, RR 16/min, weight 137.5 lbs.

Examination of the head was unremarkable except for early cataracts on both sides. Jugular venous pressure was raised to 5 cm. On auscultation, heart sounds were normal. There was a grade II/VI systolic ejection murmur at the second left intercostal area in the parasternal region. Lungs were clear. The abdomen was scarred from previous surgeries. It was soft and nontender. Bowel sounds were normal. The allograft was nontender and there was no bruit. There was moderate pitting edema of both legs extending up to the knees.

Laboratory Data

Laboratory findings are disclosed in Table 2-1. Table 2-2 shows BUN and creatinine and urinalysis over last several outpatient visits.

Radiologic Studies

Ultrasonography showed no evidence of hydronephrosis or renal artery stenosis. Isotope renogram disclosed heterogenous isotope uptake

Table 2-1. Laboratory Data

U/A	Protein 4+, blood negative, glucose 2+, no casts
CBC, platelets	Normal
PT, PTT	Normal
Bleeding time	Normal
Na 141 mEq/L, K 4.5 mEq/L, Cl 105 mEq/L, CO_2 24 mEq/L, glucose 176 mg/dl	
Ca 8.9 mg/dl, P 3.7 mg/dl, alkaline phosphatase 91 U/L	
Total protein 5.6 g/dl, albumin 2.9/dl	
Total bilirubin 0.4 mg/dl, LDH 194U/L, SGOT 35U/L	
Cholesterol 281 mg/dl, triglyceride 279 mg/dl	
24-h urine protein > 8 g	

Table 2-2. Bun, Creatinine, and U/A over Last Several Visits

Date	11/10/92	7/28/93	8/25/93	11/2/93
BUN (mg/dl)	16	20	17	37
Creatinine (mg/dl)	1.0	1.1	1.1	2.9
U/A				
Protein	Negative	Negative	Negative	4+
Blood	Negative	Negative	Negative	Negative

in right pelvis, suggesting infarction, infiltrating process, or papillary necrosis. Overall, renal function was fair to good.

DIFFERENTIAL DIAGNOSIS

Various conditions need to be differentiated in a patient with renal allograft dysfunction 10 years after transplantation (Table 2-3).

PATHOLOGY REPORT

The renal biopsy showed eight glomeruli, two of which were hyalinized. The remaining open glomeruli (Fig. 2-1) showed irregular mesangial proliferation and expansion. Capillary basement membranes were unremarkable. The interstitium showed mild fibrosis and arterioles were hyalinized. No open glomeuli were available for immunofluorescence studies. Electron microscopic examination (Fig. 2-2) showed dense deposits in all mesangial regions without deposits in peripheral loops. Reticular aggregates were present in endothelial cells (Fig. 2-3). The findings are characteristic of mesangiopathic lupus nephritis, WHO class IIB.

Table 2-3. Differential Diagnosis of Allograft Dysfunction 10 Years After Transplant

Common
  Urinary tract obstruction
  Prerenal factors, e.g., hypotension, hypovolemia, congestive cardiac failure, septicemia
  Nephrotoxic agents, e.g., cyclosporine, NSAIDs, aminoglycosides
  Chronic rejection

Infrequent
  Acute rejection mostly due to noncompliance
  Vascular event: arterial thrombosis/stenosis, venous thrombosis
  Recurrence of glomerular disease
  De novo glomerular disease

Rare
  Infection involving renal parenchyma
  Neoplasia, e.g., posttransplantation lymphoproliferative disorders (PTLD)

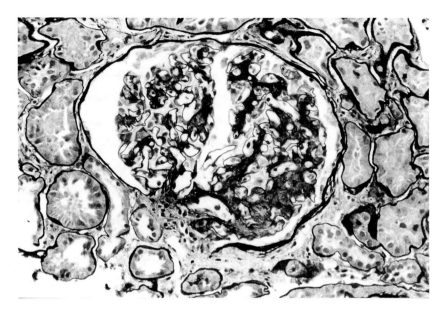

Figure 2-1. Mesangial expansion and proliferation with normal capillary basement membranes (Jones' silver stain, ×400).

DIAGNOSIS

The diagnosis was recurrence of lupus in the allograft.

DISCUSSION

In the sixties and early seventies, when experience with renal transplantation was limited, only a few experts considered lupus patients candidates for renal transplantation. It was thought that lupus, being an immune complex disease with high levels of circulating immune complexes, would recur in the allograft. Those fears were allayed when several papers reported results of transplantation in SLE comparable to other patients without SLE and insignificant recurrence rate [1]. Now, most textbooks note recurrence of lupus to be a rare phenomenon with a rate estimated to be less than 2% [2, 3, 4]. It is thought that immunosuppressive therapy keeps the recurrence rate low. The reported rarity of recurrence can be explained partly by the fact that most of the transplant centers rarely do biopsies on asymptomatic patients with stable renal function and many centers probably do not report their pa-

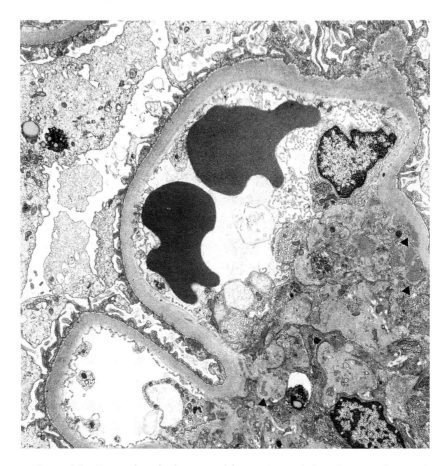

Figure 2-2. Dense deposits in mesangial area (transmission electron micrograph, ×2000).

tients with recurrence. Two centers, that use biopsy more aggressively, recently reported recurrence rates at 11% and 44%. Overall, there are only about 20 reported cases of recurrence [5, 6].

Most of the patients reported so far had mild recurrence and renal function improved promptly with increased immunosuppressive treatment [6–10]. Graft loss due to recurrence is still rare, and when it occurs, is usually within 1 year after transplant. There are no identifiable predisposing factors leading to recurrence. Positive serologies, extrarenal manifestations, duration of dialysis before transplantation, and morphologic features have poor predictive value. Recurrence has been reported with noncompliance in only two patients, suggesting that it is

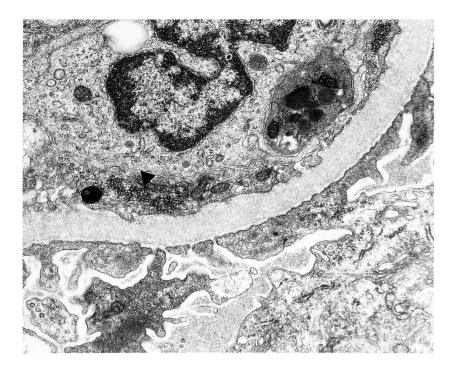

Figure 2-3. Reticular aggregate in endothelial cell cytoplasm (transmission electron micrograph, ×4900).

not a predisposing factor. However, noncompliance with immunosuppressive therapy is difficult to ascertain. Lupus can recur in cadaver as well as living-related transplant. Cyclosporine does not have any added preventive effect over azathioprine and glucocorticoids.

How, then, do we prevent or reduce the risk of recurrence? It is considered prudent to make sure that all clinical and serological manifestations of lupus are absent before transplantation. In practice, it usually means waiting for 1 year after the patient is started on dialysis. Long-term prospective studies with routine use of biopsies are necessary to answer the question definitely. However, recent data suggest that one can individualize the decision for each patient, depending on the characteristics of his/her illness. The patients with lupus can be divided into the following groups, when they present with ESRD:

1. **Clinically inactive, serologically inactive**: This is the largest group. No need to delay transplant in these patients.
2. **Clinically inactive, serologically active**: Further studies necessary. One

may wait for 1 year to transplant in this group of patients. If the disease remains silent clinically, one may transplant these patients even though serological tests are positive.

3. **Clinically active**: Clinically, the disease should be silent at least for 1 year before transplantation.
4. **Lupus with positive anticardiolipin antibody**: More experience is necessary. However, the disease should be clinically stable and there should not be any evidence of recent thrombotic episodes, because thrombosis may involve the allograft.

Our patient had a perfectly reasonable graft function for more than 10 years. On biopsy, he had recurrence of lupus (WHO classification grade IIB). Lupus serologies were negative and complements were normal. Azathioprine was increased and he was given I.V. "pulse" steroids (I.V. solumedrol 250 mg × 4) without any improvement in renal function. Unfortunately, his renal function worsened over a few months. He refused another biopsy and was started on dialysis.

As we did not perform another biopsy, it is difficult to say that his allograft was lost due to recurrence of SLE. We were reluctant to use aggressive treatment for lupus nephritis (I.V. cyclophosphamide) without another biopsy demonstrating stage III or stage IV lupus nephritis.

In conclusion, the rate of recurrence of lupus in the allograft is still unknown. It is probably more frequent than we think. Graft loss is certainly unusual. We still do not know with certainty what the predisposing factors for recurrence are. Further studies are necessary to answer these questions. It is important to make a diagnosis of recurrent lupus nephritis because graft function can be improved with increased immunosuppression.

REFERENCES

1. Ramos EL. Recurrent disease in the renal allograft. *J Am Soc Nephol* 1991;2:109–121.
2. Tisher CC. Recurrence of original disease in the transplant kidney. In: Jacobson HR, Striker GE, Klahr S, eds. *Principles and Practice of Nephrology*. Philadelphia: B. C. Dekker, Inc. 1991:852–854.
3. Ramos EL, Tilney NL, Ravenscraft MD. Clinical aspects of renal transplantation. In: Brenner BM, Rector FC, Jr. eds. *The Kidney* (4th ed.). W. B. Saunders, 1991:2361–2407.
4. Rao KV, Kjellstrand CM. Renal transplantation in specific diseases. In: Massry SG, Glassock RJ, eds. *Textbook of Nephrology* (2nd ed.). Baltimore, MD: Williams and Wilkins, 1989:1543–1550.

5. Advisory Committee to the ASG/NIH Renal Transplant Registry. Renal transplantation in congenital and metabolic diseases. *J Am Med Assoc* 1975;232:148–153.

6. Bumgardner GL, Mauer SM, Payne W, Dunn DL, Sutherland DER, Fryd DS, Ascher NL, Simmons RL, Nalavio JS. Single-center 1–15 year results of renal transplantation in patients with systemic lupus erythematous. *Transplantation* 1988;46:703–709.

7. Goss JA, Cole BR, Jendrisak MD, McCullough CS, So SKS, Windus DW, Hanto, DW. Renal transplantation for systemic lupus erythematosus and recurrent lupus nephritis: A single center experience and a review of the literature. *Transplantation* 1991;52:805–810.

8. Zara CP, Lipkowitz GS, Perri N, Sumrani N, Hong TH, Friedman EA, Butt KM. Renal transplantation and end-stage lupus nephropathy in the cyclosporine and pre-cyclosporine eras. *Transplant Proc* 1989;21:1648–1651.

9. Nyberg G, Blohme I, Persson H et al. Recurrence of SLE in transplanted kidneys: A follow-up transplant biopsy study. *Nephrol Dial Transplant* 1992;7:1116–1123.

10. Roth D, Fernandez J, Diaz A, Nery J, Burke G, Esquenazy V, Miller, J. Recurrence of lupus nephritis following renal transplantation (Abstract). *J Am Soc Nephol* 1992;2:878.

11. Lash JP. Recurrent lupus nephritis in renal allografts: More common than we think. *Kidney: A Current Survey of World Literature* 1993;2:183–186.

3

A 59-Year-Old Man with Diminished Renal Allograft Function, an Abnormal Urinalysis, and a Skin Rash

William J. Stone, Alan D. Glick, J. Harold Helderman, and Agnes Fogo

CASE PRESENTATION

History of Present Illness

A 59-year-old white man was hospitalized in December 1992 because of failing renal allograft function, hematuria, and proteinuria.

The medical history revealed 13 years of end-stage renal disease. In December 1977 he had developed fever, arthralgias, and pleural effusions. Laboratory studies showed a serum creatinine of 1.1 mg/dl, microscopic hematuria, 24-h urine protein of 2.0 g, and normal serologic tests including an ANA. He was treated with prednisone, but renal function declined. In June 1979, a renal biopsy demonstrated severe interstitial fibrosis, tubular atrophy, global and segmental glomerulosclerosis, and no evidence of immune complexes. The patient was begun on maintenance hemodialysis 3 months later.

In August 1980, he received a 3 antigen-match cadaveric renal transplant. An early episode of acute rejection responded to glucocorticoids and azathioprine. However, massive proteinuria developed in December 1980 (12.6 g/24 h). An allograft biopsy showed focal segmental glomerulosclerosis. Renal function decreased, and hemodialysis was reinstituted in November 1981. A transplant nephrectomy was performed in January 1982 in order to control hypertension. Histologic sections of the allograft again demonstrated focal segmental glomerulosclerosis.

In April 1984, he received a second cadaveric renal allograft. His renal function stabilized on prednisone and azathioprine at a serum creatinine of 1.5–1.7 mg/dl with an unremarkable urinalysis. He was able to return to work as a heavy equipment operator at a coal mine.

In December 1991, the patient developed gross hematuria and oliguria over 24 h. When he was hospitalized, laboratory tests showed a PCV of 43%, 4+ dipstick proteinuria, too numerous to count erythrocytes (RBCs) in the urine, and a serum creatinine of 3.1 mg/dl. He also gave the history of having a purpuric, lower extremity skin rash during the previous summer. Further evaluation at this time demonstrated allograft hydronephrosis. A nephrostomy produced blood clots and stones. The serum creatinine decreased to 1.4 mg/dl and he was discharged. A number of tests drawn during this admission returned following discharge. An HIV test was negative. Both IgG and IgM antibodies were positive to herpes simplex as was IgG antibody to CMV. However, cultures for CMV were negative. There was no evidence of EBV infection.

During subsequent clinic visits in the first 7 months of 1992, persistent microscopic hematuria and 1–2+ dipstick proteinuria were noted. The serum creatinine remained in normal range. A creatinine clearance in June 1992 was 84 ml/min. Immunosuppression consisted of prednisone 7.5 mg bid and azathioprine 100 mg qd. By October 1992 the serum creatinine had increased to 1.7 mg/dl, microscopic hematuria persisted, and heavy proteinuria (6.1 g/24 h) was found. His PCV was 40%. Again he complained of a purpuric rash over his lower legs during previous the summer.

He was hospitalized in December 1992 to investigate a further rise in the serum creatinine and a falling hematocrit.

Physical Examination

Vital signs: temperature 36.6°C, pulse 76/min, blood pressure 170/88 mm Hg. There were no cutaneous findings. The rash had resolved. There was no enlargement or tenderness of the renal allograft. Other than mild pedal edema, the rest of the examination was normal.

Laboratory Evaluation

The laboratory data were as follows:

Hematocrit	29%
Serum sodium	138 mEq/L

Serum potassium	4.8 mEq/L
Serum chloride	101 mEq/L
Serum bicarbonate	23 mEq/L
Serum creatinine	2.7 mg/dl
BUN	38 mg/dl
Serum albumin	2.7 g/dl
Serum calcium	8.1 mg/dl
Serum phosphate	4.3 mg/dl
Creatinine clearance	32 ml/min

Urinalysis showed 4+ blood and 4+ protein by dipstick. Microscopic examination of the urine demonstrated numerous RBCs, occasional hyaline casts, and 6–8 leukocytes (WBC) per high-power field. No RBC casts were seen. Normal tests included WBC count and differential, platelet count, RBC indices, serum urate, serum lipids, liver function tests, serum LDH, and urine culture.

Because the stool was positive for occult blood, both upper GI endoscopy and colonoscopy were performed. A Dieulafoy's ulcer of the stomach was found and cauterized. There was no further GI hemorrhage. A percutaneous biopsy of the second renal allograft was done on 9 December 1992.

Discussion of the Differential Diagnosis

Causes of renal allograft failure accompanied by hematuria and proteinuria are listed in Table 3-1. Initial historical features to be sought

Table 3-1.   Causes of Hematuria, Proteinuria, and Decreased Function in Renal Transplants

1. Obstruction of the collecting system: Blood clots, stones, fungus ball, ureteric anastomosis problems
2. Acute rejection
3. Recurrent glomerular disease: IgA nephropathy, MPGN, membranous nephropathy, anti-GBM disease, focal segmental glomerulosclerosis, diabetic glomerulosclerosis
4. Allograft glomerulopathy
5. De novo glomerulonephritis: membranous nephropathy, anti-GBM disease, postinfectious GN
6. Drug toxicity: cyclosporine, other nephrotoxic drugs
7. Thrombotic microangiopathy
8. Major arterial or venous disease in the allograft

include a list of medications (both prescribed and over the counter), the underlying cause of native kidney failure (Table 3-1), all prior allograft biopsies, any recent infections, and the use of illicit drugs. The patient should be asked about the passage of clots, gravel, or tissue per urethra. Physical examination should pay attention to the size and consistency of the allograft, signs of systemic illness (fever, rash, arthritis, ocular findings, etc.), and the presence of fluid overload or an enlarged bladder. Laboratory testing should be directed toward careful urine microscopy for dysmorphic RBCs, RBC casts, crystals, and leukocytes. A 24-h urine specimen should be collected for protein and creatinine measurements. Both ultrasonography and radionuclide scintigraphy may be helpful in ruling out renal allograft obstruction or rejection. However, percutaneous biopsy of renal transplants has been established as a very safe procedure and should be considered early in the course of patients with hematuria, proteinuria, and decreased transplant function. This is particularly true in patients who do not have an obvious cause of this syndrome and in whom laboratory testing indicates a glomerular process.

An important point is that this patient was more than 8 years posttransplant. When there is a slow loss of glomerular filtration rate (GFR) in patients who are more than 5 years posttransplant, important entities to be ruled out are urinary obstruction, allograft arterial stenosis, and cyclosporine toxicity. An abrupt drop in GFR in such a patient may mean a structural catastrophe (obstruction of vessels or collecting system), recurrent disease, a urinary leak, or acute rejection. Proteinuria of new onset in patients more than 5 years postallograft can be caused by acute rejection, chronic rejection with glomerulopathy, de novo or recurrent glomerulonephritis, or other recurrent systemic diseases (amyloid, diabetes, oxalosis) [1–3]. An approach is to follow GFR carefully, to biopsy under protocol or when GFR falls, and to pay attention to the management of hyperlipidemia. Not everyone is biopsied because chronic rejection and many types of recurrent glomerular disease are untreatable.

The Renal Biopsy

The biopsy contained 15 glomeruli, 6 of which were hyalinized. The remaining glomeruli showed segmental mesangial proliferation. Active cellular crescents (Fig. 3-1) were present in six glomeruli, with occasional areas of glomerular basement membrane breaks and fibrin. There was moderate interstitial fibrosis and tubular atrophy with a lymphoplasmacytic infiltrate confined to these areas of scarring. Arteries showed

Table 3-2. Recurrent Glomerulopathies in Renal Allografts

Type	Recurrence Rate (%)	Graft Loss (%)
Focal segmental glomerulosclerosis	20–30	30–40
Membranous nephropathy	3–7	Rare
MPGN, type I	20–30	30–40
MPGN, type II	>80	10–20
IgA nephropathy	50	10
Anti-GBM disease	12	Rare
H-S purpura	10–15	10–20
Lupus nephritis	? >10%[a]	Rare
HUS/TTP	13–25	40–50
Diabetic nephropathy	100	<5

[a]See Chapter 7 by Govani et al.
Source: Reference 3.

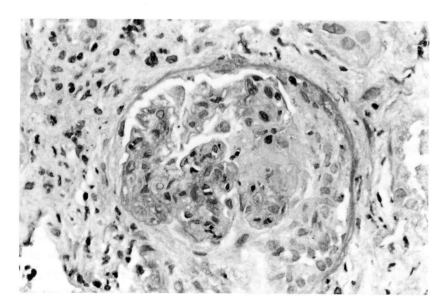

Figure 3-1. Mesangial proliferation with segmental necrosis, fibrin and early crescent formation (periodic acid–Schiff, ×430)

mild to moderate intimal fibrosis. Examination by immunofluorescence demonstrated immune deposits staining moderately for IgG, IgM, and C3 in mesangial areas and staining weakly along capillary basement membranes. By electron microscopy, large dense deposits were evident in mesangial areas with a few subendothelial deposits. The deposits were characterized by a slightly ordered pattern with microtubular substructure (Fig. 3-2).

Thus, no morphologic evidence of focal segmental glomerulosclerosis, seen in his first transplant, was evident. The interstitial and vascular intimal fibrosis was consistent with chronic rejection. In addition, there was a chronic, crescentic immune complex glomerulonephritis. The substructure of the immune deposits on electron microscopy suggested that cryoglobulinemia was the process underlying the lesions.

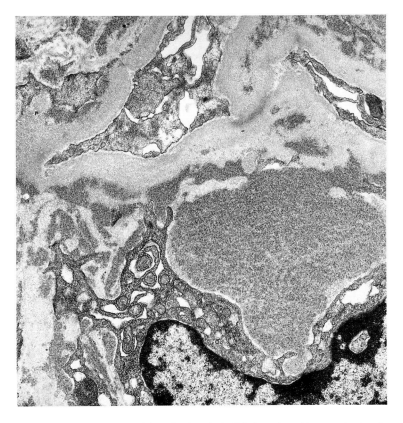

Figure 3-2. Dense mesangial and subendothelial deposits with organized, microtubular substructure (transmission electron micrograph, ×8500)

DIAGNOSIS

The diagnosis was cryoglobulinemic nephropathy in a renal allograft.

SUBSEQUENT CLINICAL COURSE

After the results of the renal biopsy were known, the serum was tested for cryoglobulins. A type III cryoglobulinemia was discovered. The cryocrit was 8.5%. The rheumatoid factor was positive in the serum at a titer greater than 1:640. The patient was hypocomplementemic with a serum C_3 of 77 mg/dl (nl 83–177), C_4 of < 8 mg/dl (nl 15–45), and a CH_{50} of < 6.7 units/ml (nl 160–400). Antibody to hepatitis C was positive by ELISA, but a hepatitis B profile was negative. ANA, c-ANCA, and RPR tests were also negative. A test for p-ANCA was positive. Immunosuppression was changed from azathioprine–prednisone to cyclosporine–prednisone to avert the potential hepatotoxicity of azathioprine. After five consecutive daily cryofiltration plasmaphereses, with 1.5 plasma volumes exchanged per treatment, the patient was discharged to outpatient plasmapheresis. The cryocrit fell to 1%. The following tests remained normal: serum bilirubin, alkaline phosphatase, and aminotransferase levels as well as prothrombin time. However, hematuria and proteinuria persisted, and the serum creatinine ranged from 1.6 to 2.2 mg/dl in early 1993. A second biopsy showed persistent crescents and more marked mesangial proliferation with immune deposits similar to the first biopsy. The patient underwent cryofiltration–plasmapheresis until April 1993. Despite this therapy and continued prednisone–cyclosporine, renal function progressively declined. A transplant nephrectomy was performed in September 1993. Examination of histologic sections of the resected allograft demonstrated chronic active rejection and progression of the crescentic immune complex glomerulonephritis, involving nearly all glomeruli. Efforts to document hepatitis C virus in renal tissue by a new immunostaining protocol failed. The patient was restarted on hemodialysis.

DISCUSSION

Case reports in transplantation become useful teaching formats if they can highlight general approaches to disease or emphasize a newly appreciated clinical relationship that will influence clinical practice. This case fulfills both criteria. First, the utility of renal biopsy is demonstrated in clarifying the disease process causing hematuria, proteinuria, and diminished GFR in a renal transplant recipient. Second, the transplant physician learns that the association of hepatitis C and cryoglobulinemia holds true for the renal allograft as well as for the native kidney [4, 5]. Late loss of allografts from cryoglobulinemia due to hepatitis C may be more frequent than is appreciated. The key will be to biopsy more transplant patients with the clinical diagnosis of "chronic rejection" or with signs of both hepatic and glomerular disease.

Both hepatitis C and cryoglobulinemia were unsuspected in this patient before the renal allograft biopsy was evaluated. He had manifested no clinical or laboratory stigmata of chronic liver disease. There were two findings attributable to cryoglobulinemia: the glomerular injury and a purpuric skin rash over the legs. The first is a very unusual but reported cause of renal transplant dysfunction [6]. The rash was probably also due to cryoglobulinemia, but this has not been confirmed by biopsy. The patient has not had a liver biopsy.

Renal involvement is usually a late feature of mixed cryoglobulinemia (type II or III) [7]. About half of the patients present with modest proteinuria and microscopic hematuria, accompanied by renal insufficiency in some patients. One-fourth have an acute nephritic picture, 20% have nephrotic syndrome, and 5% develop acute oliguric renal failure at presentation. Renal biopsy pathology shows a mesangial proliferative or membranoproliferative glomerulonephritis (MPGN), sometimes with crescents. Amorphous, eosinophilic deposits, which are PAS positive but Congo red negative, fill capillary loops. The glomerular basement membrane may appear thickened with a double contour. Immunofluorescent microscopy typically demonstrates staining with antisera to IgG, IgM, and C_3. On electron microscopy, characteristic microtubular deposits are seen in the mesangial areas, subendothelial space, and even in the capillary lumen [7, 8]. Once diagnosed, cryoglobulinemia is treated with immunosuppressive drugs and plasmapheresis, dependent on clinical severity.

Hepatitis B was implicated in the pathogenesis of mixed cryoglobulinemia (MC) in 1977 [9]. However, this infection has only explained the pathogenesis of MC in a minority of patients. With the development of serologic testing for hepatitis C virus (HCV) in recent years, an antibody to HCV has been found in about 50% of MC patients [5]. Conversely, when studying a series of consecutive patients with apparent "idiopathic" MPGN on renal biopsy, a majority had evidence of HCV infection, in contrast to patients with other renal lesions in whom hepatitis C was rare [10]. HCV may be an important cause of both and cryoglobulin-related and noncryoglobulinemic MPGN [11].

Hepatitis C is a growing problem in both dialysis and renal transplant programs. From 10% to 30% of hemodialysis patients in the United States are anti-HCV positive [12]. In a recent study from Florida, 17% of 641 renal allograft recipients were anti-HCV positive at the time of transplantation [12]. Although the authors found no effect on anti-HCV status on patient or graft survival, they recommended a pretransplant liver biopsy in anti-HCV-positive patients to stage the disease. Chronic hepatitis, progressive to cirrhosis with hepatic failure or hepatocellular carcinoma, is a worrisome feature of HCV infection [13]. Another recent study of hepatitis C in 120 Belgian renal allograft recipients documented that 14% were anti-HCV positive pretransplant [14]. After a mean posttransplant follow-up of 54 ± 28 months, all patients who were anti-HCV positive pretransplant were still positive, and five previously negative patients had become positive. Many of them had normal aminotransferase levels. There was frequent detection of HCV RNA in positive patients, indicating a persistent infection. These authors concluded that HCV infection was the main cause of liver dysfunction in renal allograft recipients [14].

Although plasmapheresis is useful in the acute setting, the best current therapy of HCV-related cryoglobulinemia may be interferon α-2a [15]. A recent controlled study of 53 such patients from Italy documented decreases in serum levels of anti-HCV, HCV RNA, cryoglobulins, rheumatoid factor, and creatinine following twice weekly injections of interferon α-2a [16]. When therapy was stopped, viremia and cryoglobulinemia recurred. When treatment was restarted, three of four patients went into a clinical, virologic, and biochemical remission.

In summary, cryoglobulinemic nephropathy related to HCV infection was a surprising finding in a patient with apparent chronic rejection, who was over 8 years post-renal-transplantation. The process was severe enough to cause loss of the renal allograft despite the absence of clinical signs of liver disease. Late manifestations of this indolent viral infection, both in the liver and kidney, are going to be a problem in end-stage renal disease patients for years to come. A high index of suspicion among dialysis and transplant physicians will be necessary to diagnose and treat HCV infection at an early stage in their patients so that irreversible organ damage will be averted.

ACKNOWLEDGMENTS

The authors thank Dr. Eleanor Ramos for permission to use Table 3-2 and Ms. Darlene Anderson for expert secretarial assistance.

REFERENCES

1. Kirkman RL, Strom TB, Weir MR et al. Late mortality and morbidity in recipients of long-term renal allografts. *Transplantation* 1982;34:347–351.

2. Braun WE. Long-term complications of renal transplantation. *Kidney Int* 1990;37:1363–1378.

3. Ramos EL. Recurrent diseases in the renal allograft. *J Am Soc Nephrol* 1991;2:109–121.

4. Agnello V, Chung RT, Kaplan LM. A role for hepatitis C virus infection in type II cryoglobulinemia. *N Engl J Med* 1992;327:1490–1495.

5. Cacoub P, Fabiani FL, Musset L et al. Mixed cryoglobulinemia and hepatitis C virus. *Am J Med* 1994;96:124–132.

6. Hiesse C, Bastuji-Garin S, Santelli G et al. Recurrent essential mixed cryoglobulinemia in renal allografts. *Am J Nephrol* 1989;9:150–154.

7. D'Amico G, Colasanti G, Ferrario F et al. Renal involvement in essential mixed cryoglobulinemia. *Kidney Int* 1989;35:1004–1014.

8. Perez GO, Pardo V, Fletcher MA. Renal involvement in essential mixed cryoglobulinemia. *Am J Kidney Dis* 1987;10:276–280.

9. Levo Y, Gorevic PD, Kassab HJ et al. Association between hepatitis B virus and essential mixed cryoglobulinemia. *N Engl J Med* 1977;296:1501–1504.

10. Yamabe H, Fukushi K, Ohsawa H et al. Hepatitis C virus (HCV) infection may be an important cause of membranoproliferative glomerulonephritis (MPGN) in Japan (Abstract). *J Am Soc Nephrol* 1993;4:291.

11. Johnson RJ, Gretch DR, Yamabe H et al. Membranoproliferative glomerulonephritis associated with hepatitis C infection. *N Engl J Med* 1993;328:465–470.

12. Roth D, Zucker K, Cirocco R et al. The impact of hepatitis C virus infection on renal allograft recipients. *Kidney Int* 1994;45:238–244.

13. Resnick RH, Koff R. Hepatitis C-related hepatocellular carcinoma. Prevalence and significance. *Arch Intern Med* 1993;153:1672–1677.

14. Goffin E, Pirson Y, Cornu C et al. Outcome of HCV infection after renal transplantation. *Kidney Int* 1994;45:551–555.

15. Levey JM, Bjornsson B, Banner B et al. Mixed cryoglobulinemia in chronic hepatitis C infection. A clinicopathologic analysis of 10 cases and review of recent literature. *Medicine* 1994;73:53–67.

16. Misiani R, Bellavita P, Fenili D et al. Interferon alfa-2a therapy in cryoglobulinemia associated with hepatitis C virus. *N Engl J Med* 1994;330:751–756.

4

A Renal Transplant Recipient Presenting 7 Years After Transplantation with Urinary Tract Obstruction and Chronic Meningitis

Keith R. Superdock and J. Harold Helderman

CASE REPORT

The patient was a 58-year-old white male from Tennessee who developed end-stage renal disease presumed secondary to analgesic nephropathy in the fall of 1984. He received a 2 haplotype living-related transplant from his sister in May 1985. His posttransplant course was complicated by an episode of acute rejection requiring treatment with intravenous solumedrol and antithymocyte serum. His serum creatinine stabilized at 1.7 mg/dl. Subsequently, he suffered from multiple medical and psychiatric illnesses including alcohol abuse and bipolar personality disorder. His chest x-rays were incidently noted to show extensive old granulomatous disease.

Two months prior to admission in 1992, he was admitted to an outside hospital with pancytopenia. His white blood cell count was 2.2 thousand per cubic millimeter, platelet count 118 thousand per cubic millimeter, and hematocrit 18% with guaiac positive stools. An upper endoscopy revealed an old healed pyloric channel ulcer. A colonoscopy revealed 3 large polyps in the sigmoid colon which were removed and found to be tubular adenomas. No clear etiology was defined for his pancytopenia.

Three days prior to admission to Vanderbilt University Hospital he was again admitted to his local hospital with low-grade fevers, an elevated GGT, pancytopenia, pyuria, fecal incontinence, and an increase in his serum creatinine from 1.7 to 2.5 mg/dl. He was transferred to Vanderbilt for further evaluation. His admission medications included azathioprine 125 mg p.o. q.h.s. and methylprednisolone 5 mg p.o. q.d.

On admission he appeared chronically ill and was mildly cushingoid but was in no acute distress. His vital signs were normal and he was afebrile. His head, lymph node, neck, cardiac, and lung exams were unremarkable. His abdomen was mildly distended with bilateral flank dullness on percussion. He had no appreciable organomegaly. A surgical scar was present in the right lower quadrant and a renal allograft was palpable. The graft was firm, nontender, and without bruits. Rectal exam was notable for decreased rectal tone and guaiac positive stool. Neurological exam was nonfocal; he was somnolent but oriented to person, place, and date.

The patient's azathioprine was discontinued. A hematologic workup for pancytopenia showed normal values for ferritin, iron, folate, and vitamin B_{12}. A bone marrow biopsy revealed no tumors or granulomata. Gastrointestinal evaluation for his liver disease, ascites, and heme positive stool was performed. An abdominal CT scan revealed marked ascites. The liver was small and had an irregular surface consistent with cirrhosis. The spleen was mildly enlarged at 13 cm. Hepatitis C antibody, hepatitis B serologies, α-fetoprotein level, ceruloplasmin, and ferritin were all within normal limits. A CEA level was mildly elevated at 9.5. Paracentesis revealed a transudate with 171 white blood cells, 88% of which were neutrophils. Cytology, as well as stains and cultures for fungus and acid fast bacilli, were negative. Upper endoscopy revealed mild esophagitis, and colonoscopy was unremarkable.

Next, the patient's elevated creatinine and pyuria were evaluated. Stains and culture of urine for acid fast bacilli were negative. A pelvic CT scan revealed a calcified mass in the collecting system of the renal allograft and caliceal dilation (Fig. 4-1). An ultrasound of the allograft revealed moderate hydronephrosis and an undetermined mass obstructing the upper pole infundibulum. A radionuclide scan of the allograft revealed poor blood flow and poor parenchymal function with an obstruction in the renal pelvis. A nephrostomy was placed into the upper pole calyces on the patient's fourth hospital day and an anterograde nephrostogram demonstrated a radiolucent 15-mm filling defect in the upper pole major infundibulum causing obstruction of all of the upper pole calyces (Fig. 4-2). Subsequently, a percutaneous nephroscopy was performed to remove the presumed nonopaque calculus. This demonstrated a shaggy, tenacious mass adherent to the wall of the in-

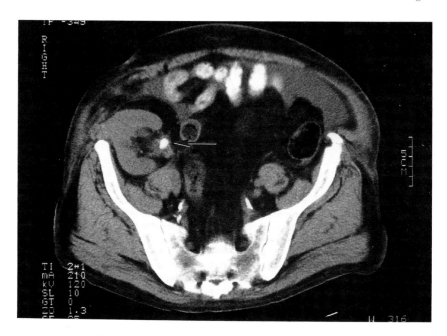

Figure 4-1. CT scan of transplant kidney. Note the calcified lesion in the renal pelvis.

fundibulum. The mass was biopsied and a partial extraction of the mass reestablished flow through the upper pole infundibulum.

A neurologic evaluation, including a lumbar puncture, was performed because of the presence of somnolence and fecal incontinence. Cerebrospinal fluid examination revealed a glucose of 42 (concomitant serum glucose was 91 mg/dl), a protein of 63 mg/dl, and a white blood cell count of 38 with 93% mononuclear cells. India ink study, cryptococcal antigen, and fungal and acid fast bacillus stains were negative.

DISCUSSION

This is a case of a patient several years after renal transplantation who presents with urinary tract obstruction and a systemic illness characterized by low-grade fevers, pancytopenia, elevated liver enzymes and ascites, altered level of consciousness, and an abnormal cerebrospinal fluid.

Urinary obstruction after renal transplantation poses unique diagnostic challenges. As the renal allograft is denervated, acute obstruction presents with the absence of symptoms of classic renal colic. Furthermore, in addition to all of the causes of obstruction that may afflict

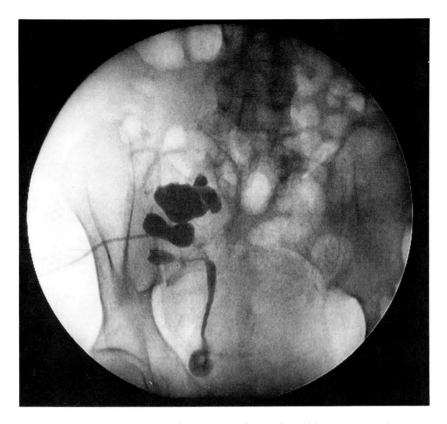

Figure 4-2. Anterograde nephrostogram of transplant kidney showing obstruction of major upper pole infundibulum.

native kidneys, the unique anatomy of the transplanted kidney, the surgical creation of a ureteroneocystostomy, and routine disruption of the normal distal ureteral vascular supply at the time of organ procurement create other potential etiologies for urinary obstruction. These etiologies include ureterovessicle obstruction due to technical error in creation of the ureteroneocystostomy; obstruction due to clots within the ureter or bladder from surgical bleeding; ureteral fibrosis and stenosis due to ischemia, inflammation, or rejection; ureteral kinking; extrinsic ureteral compression secondary to a hematoma, urinoma, or lymphocele; functional obstruction secondary to the angle of the ureterovessicle junction during bladder distension; and obstruction secondary to transplant edema [1].

The second diagnostic challenge presented here is the presence of a multiorgan system disease in a transplant patient greater than 6 months posttransplant associated with low-grade fevers and evidence of chronic meningitis. Chronic meningitis occurring in a chronically immunosuppressed transplant patient is a characteristic presentation of several potential infecting organisms. These organisms include *Cryptococcus neoformans*, *Listeria monocytogenes*, *Histoplasma capsulatum*, *Mycobacterium tuberculosis*, *Coccidiodes immitis*, *Toxoplasma gondii*, and *Nocardia* [2].

Despite the acquisition of cerebrospinal fluid, the unifying diagnosis for this patients illness was made on histologic examination of the mass extracted from the upper pole infundibulum of the transplanted kidney at the time of percutaneous nephroscopy. Hematoxylin and eosin section of the specimen showed necrotic tissue with ghosts of blood vessels and collecting tubules containing focal areas of calcification. The histopathology was compatible with necrotic renal papilla. Gomori methenamine silver and periodic acid–Schiff stains demonstrated numerous small uniform budding yeast morphologically consistent with *Histoplasma capsulatum* (Fig. 4-3).

Histoplasma capsulatum is a fungus endemic in the Mississippi and Ohio river valleys of the United States. Environmental exposure to this organism is common as evidenced by a high incidence of skin reactivity to intradermal histoplasmin antigen [3]. Disseminated disease occurs most

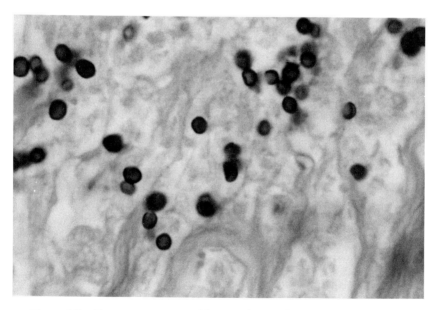

Figure 4-3. Numerous monomorphic yeast forms of *Histoplasma capsulatum* in necrotic renal papilla (Gomori's methenamine silver, ×1000).

commonly in patients with defects in cell-mediated immunity either due to age, coexistent diseases, or use of immunosuppressive agents [4]. Patients with disseminated disease typically present with fever, weight loss, weakness, fatigue, and mild respiratory symptoms [4]. In addition, organ-specific symptoms may occur in response to focal involvement of various organs [4].

Clinical manifestations of renal involvement with histoplasmosis occurs extremely uncommonly. Goodwin et al., in a review of 102 patients with disseminated histoplasmosis, noted a 40% incidence of occasional parasitized macrophages in a glomerular capillary or in the interstitial tissue of the cortex or medulla. In all cases the lesions were clinically silent with the exception of one case with destructive focal papillitis and slough into the renal pelvis [4]. Walker et al. described a case of a 56-year-old man on steroids for presumed sarcoidosis who presented with acute renal failure and postmortem evidence of papillary necrosis due to infestation with *H. capsulatum* [5]. Finally, Sridhar et al. reported a case of disseminated histoplasmosis in a renal transplant recipient who presented with a tongue ulcer and a rising serum creatinine. The patient failed to respond to presumptive therapy for rejection, and a renal transplant biopsy was obtained. The histopathology revealed medullary tissue with granulomas, central caseous necrosis, and numerous *H. capsulatum* organisms [6].

In summary, this patient was a chronically immunosuppressed Tennessee native with old granulomatous disease evident on chest radiograph who presented with urinary tract obstruction and chronic meningitis. Histopathologic diagnosis of disseminated histoplasmosis was made on percutaneous nephroscopic biopsy of an sloughed renal papilla infested with *H. capsulatum* and lodged in the upper pole infundibulum of the transplanted kidney. (Subsequent to the tissue diagnosis of disseminated histoplasmosis, the patient's cerebrospinal fluid culture also became positive for *H. capsulatum*.)

REFERENCES

1. Hunter DW, Castaneda-Zuniga WR, Coleman CC, Herrera M, Amplatz K. Percutaneous techniques in the management of urological complications in renal transplant patients. *Radiology* 1983;148:407–412.
2. Katzman M, Ellner JJ. Chronic meningitis. In Mandell GL, Douglas RG, and Bennett JE, eds. *Principles and Practice of Infectious Diseases. Third Edition.* New York: Churchill Livingstone Inc., 1990:755–762.
3. Eissenberg LG, Goldman WE: Histoplasma variation and adaptive strat-

egies for parasitism: New perspectives on histoplasmosis. *Clin Microbiol Rev* 1991;4:411–421.

4. Goodwin RA, Shapiro JL, Thurman GH, Thurman SS, Des Prez RM. Disseminated histoplasmosis: Clinical and pathologic correlations. *Medicine* 1980;59:1–33.

5. Walker JV, Baran D, Yakub YN, Freeman RB. Histoplasmosis with hypercalcemia, renal failure, and papillary necrosis—confusion with sarcoidosis. *J Am Med Assoc* 1977;237:1350–1352.

6. Sridhar NR, Tchervenkov JI, Weiss MA, Hijazi YM, First MR. Disseminated histoplasmosis in a renal transplant patient: A cause of renal failure several years following transplantation. *Am J Kidney Dis* 1991;17:719–721.

5

A Renal Transplant Recipient with Fever and Gastrointestinal Bleeding

Stephen Dummer and David Van Buren

A 69-year-old woman received a cadaveric renal transplant 15 years earlier after developing renal failure from the administration of iodinated intravenous contrast. Recently, she had developed chronic rejection with creatinine values ranging from 2.5 to 3.0 mg/dl. She had suffered a myocardial infarction 29 years ago and had hypertension and gout. Over the past 6 months she had developed anemia and required transfusions on two occasions. No site of blood loss was detected. The anemia was ascribed to inadequate red blood cell production resulting from chronic renal dysfunction and the marrow-suppressive effects of azathioprine therapy. One month earlier she had been admitted to the hospital with low-grade fever, cough, arthralgia, myalgias, and vomiting. Her hematocrit was 22 vol%, but her stools were guaiac negative. She was febrile to 102.4°F. Transfusions were given and she was treated with broad-spectrum antibacterial therapy for bronchitis. Her fever fell to 100°F, and she was discharged home.

The patient was now readmitted with recurrent symptoms of fever, vomiting and cough with episodes of lightheadedness. She was febrile to 99.7°F, her pulse was 82, respiration rate 20, and blood pressure 128/62. The head and neck exam was unremarkable. The chest was clear and there were no heart murmurs. Her abdomen was diffusely tender but without rebound; no masses were noted. Her stool was guaiac negative. No edema or cyanosis was noted. The patients medications included azathioprine 25 mg/day, prednisone 5 mg bid, allopurinol 100 mg daily, diltiazem 60 mg tid, clonidine 0.1 bid, rocalcitrol 2.5 mg weekly, and isordil 60 mg tid.

LABORATORY EXAM

The results were sodium 130, potassium 4.8, chloride 94, bicarbonate 26, glucose 88, BUN 88, creatinine 3.0, white blood cell count 3700, hemoglobin 7.3, hematocrit 1.0, and platelets 201,000; the white cell differential had 88% neutrophils, 8% lymphocytes, 2% monocytes, and 2% eosinophil. The chest radiograph showed a few calcific densities consistent with old granulomatous disease and a faint infiltrate at the right costophrenic angle. No free-flowing fluid was detected by decubitus chest radiographs.

HOSPITAL COURSE

The patient was transfused with two units of blood and begun on intravenous erythromycin as coverage for presumed community-acquired pneumonia. Over the next few days the low-grade fevers persisted, but the patient's serum creatinine fell to 1.9 with hydration. The syncopal episodes cleared and were thought to be due to volume depletion. Routine cultures of blood, urine, and sputum were negative. One week into the hospitalization, the patient developed brisk gastrointestinal bleeding with melanotic stools. At upper gastrointestinal endoscopy, an erythematous mass was noted on the medial wall of the duodenum. A biopsy of this lesion showed numerous histiocytes. No organisms were seen on special stains. Colonoscopy to the level of the cecum showed dark guaiac positive stool but was otherwise normal. The patient continued to bleed and required seven more units of blood. A tagged red blood cell scan disclosed a bleeding site in the small bowel and, on follow-up, arteriogram extravasation of dye was seen in the proximal jejunum. On the 13th day of hospitalization a laparotomy was performed. A mass was found in the proximal small bowel. It appeared to arise inside the lumen but extended through the wall of the bowel and indented the C-loop of the duodenum. Ten inches of involved jejunum was resected and the uninvolved ends were reanastomosed. On histology, granulomatous inflammation was seen that involved the full thickness of the bowel wall with mucosal ulceration. Numerous yeast forms consistent with *Histoplasma capsulatum* were identified by silver stain. After the operation, amphotericin B was administered and the patient recuperated slowly over the next $2\frac{1}{2}$ weeks. She had no more bleeding. Complement fixation titers for histoplasma were positive with a titer of 1:8, but *H. capsulatum* did not grow from the jejunal specimen. The patient received 330 mg amphotericin B in the hospital and was then discharged on 30 mg intravenously three times a week via a Hickman catheter. A total dose of 1.5 g was planned, to be followed by a prolonged course of oral ketoconazole. The patient developed sepsis from her Hickman catheter about 1 month after discharge and died at an outlying hospital.

DISCUSSION

The diagnosis of gastrointestinal histoplasmosis was made in this patient after massive gastrointestinal bleeding led to aggressive evaluation and surgical treatment. It is likely that this disease had been smoldering for some months, but the intermittent nature of the bleeding and the failure to detect occult blood in the stool delayed the diagnosis. After resection of the involved area of bowel and treatment with amphotericin B, the patient improved steadily but unfortunately succumbed to a catheter-related bacteremia.

Histoplasma capsulatum is a pathogenic fungus of worldwide distribution. It is particularly prevalent in areas of the midwestern and southeastern United States bordering the Ohio and Mississippi river valleys. The organism is present in soil, and humans acquire infection through inhalation. In some endemic areas, over 90% of individuals show evidence of infection with the organism by skin test reactivity. The generally low virulence of the fungus is shown by the disparity between this high rate of actual infection and the low rate of serious infection that reaches medical attention. Most infections are asymptomatic or cause mild self-limited respiratory disease. Chronic apical pulmonary disease that is somewhat similar to apical tuberculosis may occasionally be seen but is usually confined to individuals with chronic lung diseases, particularly emphysema. Disseminated disease has been estimated to occur in only 1:100,000 or fewer of all infected individuals but is certainly becoming more common because of the AIDS epidemic. Most patients with disseminated disease have underlying medical conditions causing defects of cell-mediated immunity that predispose them to dissemination.

The frequency of histoplasmosis at two renal transplant centers was 0.4% and 2.1% [1, 2]. The higher rate was from a center in Indiana where communitywide outbreaks of histoplasmosis occurred. Vanderbilt is in a highly endemic area for histoplasmosis. A recent review of the Vanderbilt experience with histoplasmosis in the renal transplant population over the last decade has turned up 10 definite cases. This represents slightly less than 1% of the patients at risk. Seven of these patients had extra pulmonary or disseminated disease. All but one of these cases occurred 2 or more years after transplantation. One patient with relapsing histoplasma meningitis died of the disease. Relapses after apparently successful treatment were seen in four patients.

Symptoms of disseminated histoplasmosis are most often nonspecific and include weight loss, chronic fever, and generalized malaise [3]. Hepatomegaly, splenomegaly, and lymphadenopathy are found in a significant minority (20–30%) of patients. The most common laboratory findings are anemia, leukopenia, and thrombocytopenia; these abnormalities increase in frequency with increased severity of the disease. Detection of *Histoplasma capsulatum* outside of the lung in a symptomatic patient is almost always an indication of disseminated disease. The gastrointestinal tract may be involved anywhere from the oral cavity to the rectum [4, 5]. Nodular and ulcerative lesions are seen and may mimic carcinoma or inflammatory bowel disease. Symptoms of nausea, vomiting, diarrhea, and abdominal pain are common. Complete bowel ob-

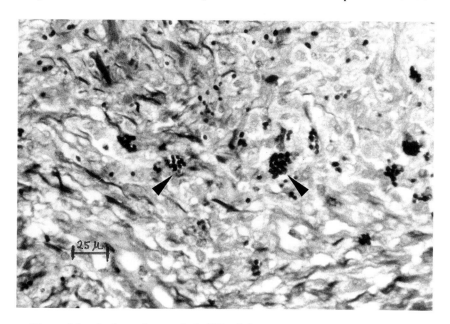

Figure 5-1. A photomicrograph (×500) of the resected jejunal tissue stained with methenamine silver shows clusters of small yeast forms of *Histoplasma capsulatum* (arrows).

struction and perforation with generalized peritonitis have both been described.

The current case is somewhat unusual in that clinically apparent disease was restricted to a localized area of the small bowel. Cappell et al. [4] have recently collected 77 cases of primary gastrointestinal histoplasmosis from the world literature and noted that most cases represented diagnostic enigmas. In one-third, the diagnosis was made only at autopsy. Clearly, gastrointestinal histoplasmosis is a diagnostic consideration when a chronic, debilitating disease with abdominal symptoms occurs in a transplant patient, particularly if the transplant patient lives in an endemic region.

The diagnosis of histoplasmosis can be made by culture, tissue sections, and examination of body fluids for histoplasma antigen [6]. Culture is highly specific but slow. Cultures may take 4–8 weeks to turn positive. For this reason it is important to obtain a histological diagnosis whenever possible. In the current case, the pathology of the jejunal lesion itself made the diagnosis. The bone marrow is a useful site to biopsy when there is no apparent lesion to biopsy. Urine, blood, and spinal fluid also can be analyzed for histoplasma antigen by Dr. Joseph Wheat's laboratory in Indianapolis, Indiana. The test is specific. The sensitivity is about 90% for urine samples and 50% for blood specimens.

Disseminated histoplasmosis is treated either with intravenous amphotericin B or oral azoles (ketoconazole or itraconazole). In immunocompromised hosts, the initial treatment should be with amphotericin B, and a course of 2 g or more is usually recommended. In selected patients it may be possible to switch to less toxic azole therapy after an initial period of amphotericin treatment. Long-term prophylaxis against relapse with oral antifungals has not been studied but might be considered in patients thought to be at high risk.

REFERENCES

1. Wheat LJ, Smith EJ, Sathapatayavongs B et al. Histoplasmosis in renal allograft recipients. *Arch Intern Med* 1983;143:703–707.
2. Davies SF, Sarosi GA, Peterson PK et al. Disseminated histoplasmosis in renal transplant recipients. *Am J Surgery* 1979;137:686–691.
3. Goodwin RA, Jr, Shapiro JL, Thurman GH, et al. Disseminated histoplasmosis: Clinical and pathologic correlations. *Medicine* 1980;59:1–27.
4. Cappell MS, Mandell W, Grimes MM et al. Gastrointestinal histoplasmosis. *Dig Dis Sci* 1988;33:353–360.

5. Perez CA, Sturim HS, Kochoukos NT et al. Some clinical radiographic features of gastrointestinal histoplasmosis. *Surgery* 1965;86:482–487.
6. Wheat LJ, Kohler RB, Tewau RP. Diagnosis of disseminated histoplasmosis by detecting of *Histoplasma capsulatum* antigen in serum and urine specimens. *N Engl J Med* 1986;314:83–88.

6

Fever, Hematuria, Vomiting, and Constipation in a Young Man with a Poorly Functioning Renal Allograft

William J. Stone

CLINICAL PRESENTATION

A 33-year-old white man from rural Virginia received an HLA-identical renal transplant from his sister. Although the graft functioned well initially, acute rejection ensued. He developed fever and graft tenderness. A rising serum creatinine and an abnormal radionuclide renogram were noted. Parenteral methylprednisolone and graft irradiation were administered, but the serum creatinine remained at 7.1–7.7 mg/dl. He was discharged after 7 weeks on prednisone 40 mg and azathioprine 100 mg daily.

One month later he was hospitalized because of fever, nausea, vomiting, headache, dysuria, and throat soreness. Hemodialysis was reinstituted because of worsened renal function. A 12% peripheral blood eosinophilia was present. Symptoms quickly abated. Prednisone dosage was decreased to 20 mg daily. Azathioprine was continued at 100 mg daily.

Two months after the transplant he was again hospitalized. Fever, malaise, nausea, vomiting, and diarrhea were present. Symptoms were attributed to graft rejection, and it was removed. Pathologic examination of the graft demonstrated organized thrombi resulting in massive necrosis of both cortex and medulla. Peripheral blood eosinophilia averaged 14% during the admission. Gastrointestinal symptoms were not prominent in the postoperative period. He was discharged after 2 weeks on a regimen including prednisone 10 mg daily. Azathioprine therapy was stopped.

Within 2 weeks, the patient again developed fever, chills, and vomiting. He also had gross hematuria and constipation. He had decided on his own to stop taking prednisone. Upon hospitalization there were no abnormal physical findings.

LABORATORY EVALUATION

The laboratory data were as follows:

Hematocrit	29%
WBC	7000 cells/µl
Neutrophils	16%
Lymphocytes	27%
Eosinophils	53%
Monocytes	4%
Platelet count	149,000/µl
BUN	48 mg/dl
Serum creatinine	14.5 mg/dl
Total serum protein	5.6 g/dl
Serum albumin	3.1 g/dl

The following tests were normal or negative: serum glucose, serum electrolytes, liver function studies, serum calcium and phosphorus, blood, and urine cultures, spinal fluid examination, stool for parasites, and radiographs of the chest and abdomen. A baseline serum cortisol level was normal as was the response of the serum cortisol to ACTH.

HOSPITAL COURSE

The patient first had cystoscopy to evaluate hematuria. An abnormal-appearing area was seen at the previous ureterovesical anastomosis. It was not actively bleeding and showed only granulation tissue when biopsied. Cefazolin and tobramycin were given. Although glucocorticoids were started to cover potential adrenal insufficiency, these agents were stopped when the normal serum cortisol values returned. Persistence of the striking peripheral blood eosinophilia (3500 cells/μl) caused examination of both a duodenal aspirate and more stool specimens. The former was unrevealing, but the latter demonstrated filariform larvae of *Strongyloides stercoralis* (Fig. 6-1). He was sent home after receiving 7 days of oral thiabendazole, 3.0 daily, and on no immunosuppression.

In the follow-up period, the patient had no recurrence of strongyloidiasis as monitored by regular stool examinations. The course of his antibody response to the parasite is shown in Figure 6-2. The patient subsequently was able to receive a second renal transplant from another sister and has done well. There was no evidence of strongyloidiasis at 5 years follow-up (Fig. 6-2).

DISCUSSION

The parasitic roundworm, *Strongyloides stercoralis*, is endemic in parts of the United States and in a large portion of the rest of the world. It causes gastrointestinal illness in normal human hosts and may be harbored for more than 30 years in a relatively symbiotic relationship with

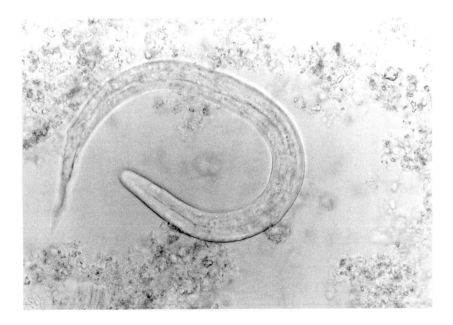

Figure 6-1. Filariform larva of *Strongyloides stercoralis* (×400).

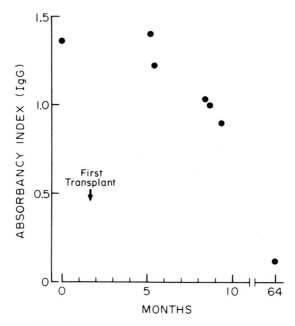

Figure 6-2.   Serial levels of serum IgG antibodies directed against *S. stercoralis* antigens. Analyses were done on frozen stored samples from the patient under discussion.

the host. The life cycle of *Strongyloides stercoralis* is similar to hookworm. Both adult worms and larvae of *Strongyloides stercoralis* can survive in soil and in certain animal reservoirs. In the soil, noninvasive larvae become potentially invasive (filariform). These filariform larvae can penetrate human skin on contact. A syndrome of cutaneous larval migrans results. The burrowing larvae gain access to the vasculature and are taken to the lungs and other organs. Eventually, they reach the upper gastrointestinal tract. The larvae mature into parthenogenetic adult females which live in the duodenal mucosa. Eggs are produced and yield noninvasive larvae (rhabditiform), which are expelled in the stool to complete the cycle.

However, compromised human hosts develop a much more serious illness when infected with this parasite. There is an augmentation of worm burden in the lungs and intestine. Additionally, transformation of noninvasive rhabditiform larvae to filariform larvae occurs in the host's GI tract. Bacteremia, peritonitis, pneumonia, meningitis, and urinary tract infection result from bacteria brought along by the larvae burrowing through the intestine. Typically, gut flora such as *Escherichia coli, Klebsiella pneumoniae, Bacteroides fragilis,* and *Streptococcus faecalis* are cultured from the patient's blood, urine, peritoneal fluid, or cerebrospinal fluid. The clinician is confronted with a bewildering illness involving multiple organ systems and positive bacterial cultures. Everything may be attributed to "sepsis." Pulmonary syndromes can appear to be carcinoma, abscess, hemorrhage, asthma, or respiratory failure as well as various types of pneumonia. Nausea, vomiting, diarrhea, GI hemorrhage, ileus, abdominal pain and tenderness, dehydration, malnutrition, and perianal ulcers can mislead physicians into considering viral gastroenteritis, peptic ulcer disease, carcinoma, inflammatory bowel disease (Crohn's disease or ulcerative colitis), antibiotic colitis, and a host of other erroneous diagnoses. CNS manifestations include meningeal signs, mental status changes, convulsions, stupor, and coma. CSF cultures may be positive. Brain abscess, other opportunistic infections, CNS lymphoma, stroke, seizure disorders, or other misdiagnoses are often considered first. The urticarial rash and pruritus may be subtle, ignored, or attributed to the many drugs being given to transplant recipients. These varied clinical manifestations of systemic strongyloidiasis (Table 6-1) lead to misdiagnoses, inappropriate therapy, and a fatal outcome in more than 50% of patients.

Diagnosis

The biggest problems in strongyloidiasis are considering the diagnosis of this infection in the first place and then being persistent in

Table 6-1 Symptoms of Opportunistic Strongyloidiasis

Pulmonary	Central nervous system
Cough	Meningeal signs
Chest pain	Mental status changes
Dyspnea/wheezing	Stupor, coma
Hemoptysis	Seizures
Cyanosis	
Gastrointestinal	Constitutional
Abdominal pain/distention	Fever, chills
Nausea/vomiting/anorexia	Malaise
Diarrhea	Weakness
Hematemesis/melena	Weight loss
Perianal ulcers	Shock
Cutaneous	
Creeping eruption	
Urticaria	
Pruritus	
Rash	
Edema	

looking for the parasite. In an organ transplant recipient with a pulmonary, GI, bacteremic, and/or meningitic illness, it is important to look at multiple specimens of stool and duodenal aspirate for the larvae. Invasive larvae are highly mobile in fresh specimens. They have a whip-like action and are easily seen under low-power microscopy. If there is pulmonary involvement, fresh sputum specimens should also be carefully examined for larvae. Serendipitous diagnoses are made about half the time in cases of opportunistic strongyloidiasis. Tests to exclude cancer (sputum Pap smears, biopsy of bronchial lesions, or GI ulcers), inflammatory bowel disease, or other opportunistic pathogens instead reveal larvae of *Strongyloides stercoralis*. Alert microbiology technicians have noticed serpentine tracking of bacteria on sputum cultures or stool cultures. These tracks are caused by filariform larvae spreading bacteria as they crawl. One technician in our medical center correctly identified the pathogen by performing microscopy on a mucoid stool sent for occult blood testing. Obviously, serendipitous diagnosis is best avoided by being aware of the intricacies of the manifestations of this infection.

Tests that cannot be relied on to diagnose strongyloidiasis are peripheral blood eosinophilia (glucocorticoid therapy may suppress this) and single examinations of stool or upper GI aspirates. Two-thirds of parasitized renal transplant recipients have less than 10% peripheral blood eosinophilia. Additionally, there is only a 25% chance of finding the organism in one stool specimen from a patient with proven strongyloidiasis. Multiple specimens must be scanned by trained observers to make the diagnosis (Table 6-2).

Reliable antibody tests have been developed by Genta and co-work-

Table 6-2   Identification of *Strongyloides stercoralis* in 30 Renal Transplant Recipients

	Initial Diagnosis	All Specimens
Stool	25	32
Sputum for cytology	6	9
Duodenal aspirate	3	7
Urine	2	3
Bronchoscopic aspirate	2	3
Peritoneal fluid	1	1
Wound/skin	0	2
Blind loop fluid	0	1
Unknown	1	1
Autopsy	2	2
	42 episodes	61 identifications

ers. Applying both ELISA (IgG) and RAST (IgE) tests to nine renal transplant recipients with strongyloidiasis from this center, positive results were demonstrated in eight of them (89%), as shown in Figure 6-2 for the patient under discussion. Unfortunately, these tests are not widely available. Both antibody testing and stool examinations should be routinely applied to patients from endemic areas who are on transplant waiting lists. Positive tests must result in antihelminthic therapy to the patient before he is transplanted. Follow-up testing has to be performed as well to assure eradication of this parasite.

Therapy

The standard therapy of systemic strongyloidiasis in organ transplant patients has involved thiabendazole in prolonged and repeated courses. This drug is effective against both larvae and adult worms. Treatment is begun with 25 mg/kg of thiabendazole by mouth twice daily for 3–7 days. Thiabendazole may also be administered by rectum. Adjunctive therapy with standard antibiotics is given as positive cultures would indicate. Antibiotic therapy alone will not eradicate these secondary bacterial infections unless antihelminthic therapy is also given. Cambendazole, mebendazole, and pyrvinium pamoate are alternative oral antihelminthics. A veterinary drug, ivermectin, has been also reported to be effective in small numbers of normal hosts with this parasitism. Cyclosporine has been useful in treating an animal model of strongyloidiasis, *Strongyloides ratti* infection of rodents. The wide usage of cyclosporine in human organ transplantation may be responsible for the recent decrease in cases of strongyloidiasis at our center. A parenteral drug proven effective against strongyloidiasis is still a great need. Whatever type of therapy is given, vigilance to assure eradication of the parasite is the major factor determining a good outcome. Repeat courses of antihelminthics are often required. Removal of infected reservoirs (such as household pets) in the patient's environment may also be helpful. Another critical factor appears to be the reduction of immunosuppressive drugs, especially glucocorticoids, to the lowest possible doses. New information suggests that glucocorticoids may increase amounts of ecdysteroids in the patient's body. These substances send strong molting signals to noninvasive rhabditiform larvae, which then transform to invasive filariform larvae in the GI tract. Although the data are preliminary, most patients, who developed fulminant strongyloidiasis after only a few days of steroid therapy, received large doses of methylprednisolone for acute transplant rejection, as did the patient under discussion.

ACKNOWLEDGMENTS

Dr. Robert M. Genta performed the antibody determinations, and Mrs. Darlene Anderson provided expert secretarial assistance.

REFERENCES

1. DeVault GA, King JW, Rohr MS et al. Opportunistic infections with *Strongyloides stercoralis* in renal transplantation. *Rev Infect Dis* 1990;12:653–671.
2. Genta RM. Global prevalence of strongyloidiasis: Critical review with epidemiologic insights into the prevention of disseminated disease. *Rev Infect Dis* 1989;11:755–767.
3. Genta RM, Douce RW, Walzer PD. Diagnostic implications of parasite-specific immune responses in immunocompromised patients with strongyloidiasis. *J Clin Microbiol* 1986;23:1099–1103.
4. Genta RM. Dysregulation of strongyloidiasis: A new hypothesis. *Clin Microbiol Rev* 1992;5:345–355.
5. Morgan JS, Schaffner W, Stone WJ. Opportunistic strongyloidiasis in renal transplant recipients. *Transplantation* 1986;42:518–524.
6. Stone WJ, Schaffner W. Strongyloides infections in transplant recipients. *Sem Resp Infect* 1990;5:58–64.

7

Pulmonary Cavity and Skin Lesions in a Renal Transplant Patient

Mahendra V. Govani, Agnes Fogo,
and J. Harold Helderman

CASE PRESENTATION

History of Present Illness

A 52-year-old Caucasian man was admitted on 10 August 1993 for a transplant kidney biopsy because of rise in creatinine (from 1.7 to 2.4 mg/dl) and mild proteinuria. He had a 1A, 1B matched living-related kidney transplant in March 1989 for end-stage renal disease (ESRD) from autosomal dominant polycystic kidney disease (ADPKD). His creatinine typically was between 1.7 and 1.9 mg/dl. Over the last 7 months before admission, urine dipstix showed mild proteinuria intermittently. Four months before admission, 24-h urinary protein excetion was 590 mg and serum creatinine was 2.1 mg/dl; it increased to 2.4 mg/dl 10 days before admission. While he was in the hospital, he wanted to "sort out" what he called a few other "minor" problems:

1. A small painless lesion on his right forearm noted for the last 2–3 months. It was gradually increasing in size.
2. A few small elevated skin lesions on his forehead. A similar lesion was frozen about a year ago by a dermatologist in Chattanooga.
3. Mild pain on medial aspect of left knee after he twisted it a day before admission.

Eight months before admission, diabetes mellitus was diagnosed and he was started on a diabetic diet. Four months before admission, he developed vague joint pains especially in the knees and ankles and his uric acid was high. A clinical diagnosis of gout was made, probenecid was started, and his joint pains disappeared over a few weeks. There was no history of cough, chest pain, dyspnea, fever, headache, photophobia, confusion, gait disturbance, nausea, vomiting, or loss of weight. He was on cyclosporine 100 mg bid, azathioprine 100 mg qhs, prednisone 5 mg bid, atenolol 50 mg qd, isradipine 2.5 mg bid, and probenecid 500 mg bid.

Physical Examination

Vital signs: temperature 98.2 °F, BP 130/70 mm Hg, pulse 55/min and regular, and RR 16/min.

The patient weighed 58.4 kg and had mild cushingoid facies. He had a few small elevated lesions on the forehead. His upper extremities were mildly bruised. There was a small, 2–3-cm, irregular, nontender, immobile nodule on the volar aspect of right forearm. Examination of heart and lungs was unremarkable. Abdomen was soft and nontender. Left kidney was palpable and nontender. The renal allograft was nontender and there was no bruit. Bowel sounds were normal. Examination of the central nervous system was normal. There was no neck stiffness, and Kernig's sign was negative. Fundus examination revealed grade I–II hypertensive changes. There was mild tenderness on the medial aspect of the left knee and movements of the left knee were slightly restricted. Legs were nonedematous.

Laboratory Data

Laboratory values are presented in Table 7-1. Table 7-2 shows BUN and creatinine over the last several visits.

Radiologic Studies

Radiologic findings are presented in Table 7-3.

EARLY HOSPITAL COURSE

Transplant renal biopsy was done on the day of admission. On the second day, he developed swelling of the left knee and his pain got worse. Orthopedic referral was made. The knee was aspirated. Synovial fluid

Table 7-1. Laboratory Values

CBC, platelets	Normal
PT, PTT	Normal
Bleeding time	Normal

Na 143 mEq/L, K 5.2 mEq/L, Cl 100 mEq/L, CO_2 29 mEq/L, sugar 330 mg/dl
Ca 9.6 mg/dl, P 3.3 mg/dl, alkaline phosphatase 54 U/L
Total protein 6.6 g/dl, alb 3.9 g/dl
Bilirubin 0.6 mg/dl, SGOT 13 U/L, LDH 333 U/L
TG 447 mg/dl, chol 293 mg/dl
CysA level 152 ng/ml

24-h urine protein	3/30/93	590 mg
	8/10/93	320 mg
Cyclosporine level	<174 ng/ml from July 1992 to admission day	

Table 7-2. BUN and Creatinine Values

Date	3/30/93	7/20/93	7/30/93	8/10/93
BUN (mg/dl)	43	51	53	50
Creatinine (mg/dl)	1.7	2.1	2.4	2.2

Table 7-3. Radiologic Findings

Ultrasound kidney allograft	No evidence of hydronephrosis, stone, or perinephric fluid collection.
Isotope renogram	Good function, no change from last study dated 3/89; peak 6 min, 56% washout
CXR (Fig. 7-1)	Well-defined thin-walled cavitary lesion in the right lower lobe; no acute infiltrates are identified.
CT scan of chest (Fig. 7-2)	Large, 2.5 cm in axial diameter, thin-walled cavity in the superior segment of the right lower lobe; no evidence of fluid collection in the cavity; no acute infiltrates; calcified right hilar and azygous lymph nodes.

was hemorrhagic and there were no crystals. Meniscal injury was suspected. Plain x-ray films and MRI of the knee were consistent with the meniscal injury. His knee was splinted and it improved after a few days. Skin lesions on the forehead were biopsied by a dermatologist. Excision biopsy of the skin nodule was also performed 2 days after admission. Skin tests with PPD, candida antigen, and mumps antigen were negative. The patient was unable to produce adequate amount of sputum

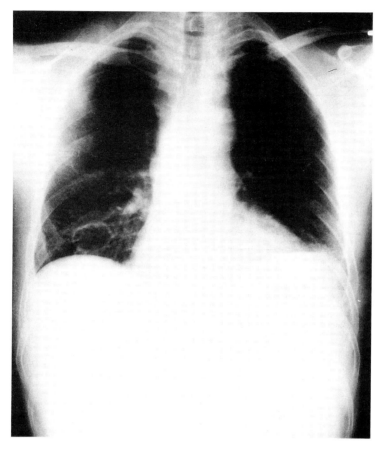

Figure 7-1. PA view of chest demonstrates a thin walled cavity in the right lower lobe.

for microscopy and culture. Various tests for cryptococcosis, blastomycosis, and histoplasmosis were ordered. He was started on an oral hypoglycemic agent for his diabetes, and his glucose levels were reasonable in the hospital.

PATHOLOGY REPORTS

The renal biopsy (Fig. 7-3) contained 17 glomeruli, 3 of which were hyalinized. The remaining glomeruli were unremarkable. The tubulointerstitium showed alternating areas of fibrosis and tubular atrophy

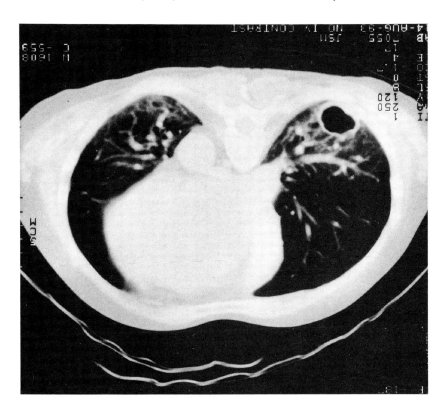

Figure 7-2. CT scan of chest reveals a cavity in the superior segment of the right lower lobe without any fluid collection.

with intervening intact tubules. Arterioles showed mild hyalinization. Immunofluorescence and electron microscopic studies were unremarkable. The pattern of interstitial fibrosis, although not diagnostic, is suggestive of chronic cyclosporine nephrotoxicity.

The skin biopsy (Fig. 7-4) revealed fat necrosis with marked acute inflammation, extending deep into subcutaneous tissues, suggesting possible panniculitis. Special stains revealed numerous mucin and methanamine silver positive yeast forms, consistent with Cryptococcus.

DIAGNOSES

The diagnoses were disseminated cryptococcosis, chronic cyclosporine toxicity, and meniscal injury of the left knee.

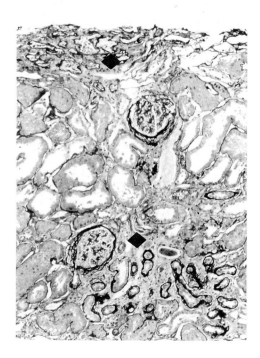

Figure 7-3. Alternating zones of interstitial fibrosis and tubular atrophy (asterisks) with intervening preserved tubules (Jones' silver stain, ×130).

LATE HOSPITAL COURSE

Lumbar puncture, done to rule out central nervous system involvement, was negative. Test for cryptococcal antigen in blood was positive in the undiluted specimen. The patient was started on oral fluconazole. His cyclosporine dose was reduced and he was discharged home with early follow-up appointment.

DISCUSSION

We will limit our discussion to the main diagnosis of disseminated cryptococcosis.

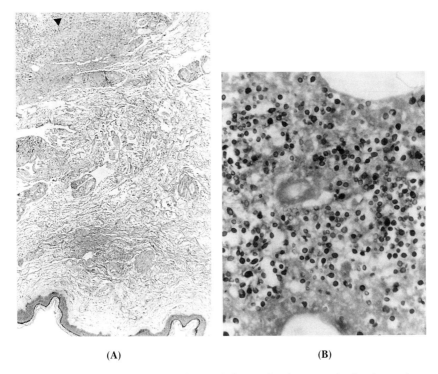

(A)   (B)

Figure 7-4. (*A*) Fat necrosis and acute inflammation is present in the deep subcutaneous tissue (arrowhead) (hematoxylin and eosin, ×70). (*B*) Numerous silver staining yeast forms are present in the area of necrosis (methenamine silver stain, ×400).

Introduction

Cryptococcosis, caused by the fungus *Cryptococcus neoformans*, is an important infection of the immunocompromised host [1–3]. The fungus reproduces by budding and forms round organisms 4–6 μm in diameter with a thick distinctive polysaccharide capsule. Inhalation of aerosolized yeast is necessary for the development of human infection. *C. neoformans* is commonly found in soil contaminated with pigeon droppings. However, history of exposure to pigeons is uncommon. There is no evidence to suggest human-to-human or animal-to-human transmission, nor are there reports of epidemics or highly endemic areas. Infection is rare among children. Adult males are twice as likely to get infection as adult females. Laboratory personnel working with the fungus are at no increased risk.

In approximately 70% of patients, a predisposing condition with impaired cell-mediated immunity is found (Table 7-4). Neutropenia and

Table 7-4. Predisposing Conditions for Cryptococcosis

Immunosuppressive therapy for transplantation
Lymphoreticular neoplasms
Acquired immunodeficiency syndrome (AIDS)
Immunosuppressive therapy for other conditions, e.g., rheumatoid arthritis
? Diabetes mellitus
? Sarcoidosis
? Job's syndrome (recurrent infections and IgE hypergammaglobulinemia)
? Low-dose methotrexate therapy for chronic arthritis

hypogammaglobulinemia are not reported to be predisposing conditions. In a transplant patient, cryptococcosis, when it occurs, usually manifests 6 months after transplant. In patients with acquired immunodeficiency syndrome (AIDS), cryptococcosis is more common, of more severe nature, and difficult to cure than in the transplant population.

Pathogenesis

Initial infection in the lung is almost always silent and resolves spontaneously. However, hematogenous spread occurs during this silent phase and organisms lodge at distant sites. The fungus has a particular tropism for the central nervous system (CNS) where it seeds especially in the perivascular areas of cortical gray matter and basal ganglia. There is little inflammatory reaction against these organism at these CNS sites, whereas there is marked granulomatous response in the lung. Basilar arachnoiditis is the feature of chronic CNS infection.

Clinical Features (Table 7-5)

Meningoencephalitis: It is the most common clinical manifestation of cryptococcosis [4]. Death is inevitable in untreated cases; however, it may take 2 weeks to several years. The onset is insidious and symptoms may wax and wane for a long time before the patient seeks attention or the diagnosis is suspected. Our patient's only symptom was his skin nodule. Lumbar puncture was normal, and although cryptococcal antigen was positive in undiluted serum, it was negative in cerebrospinal fluid (CSF). We believe that cryptococcosis was in the very early phase in his case and he was fortunate that he was admitted to the hospital for renal biopsy where his "minor" problems were investigated, before CNS involvement occured.

Pulmonary cryptococcosis: Lung infection is common and may be the only site of infection. However, the patients are mostly symptomless

Table 7-5. Clinical Features of Cryptococcosis

Meningoencephalitis	
Manifestation	Frequency
Headache	67%
Nausea and vomiting	20%
Fever	50%
Neck stiffness	20%
Papilledema	33%
Cranial nerve palsies	25%
Other uncommon features	
Staggering gait	
Confusion	
Blurred vision	
Personality changes	
Seizure	
Coma	
Pulmonary Cryptococcosis	
Chest pain	40%
Cough	20%
Skin lesions	10%
Bone lesions	4%
Other rare manifestations	
Endocarditis, pericarditis, peritonitis, hepatitis, renal abscess, prostatitis, endophthalmitis, and orchitis	

like this patient. When symptoms do occur, dry cough and chest pain are the commonest. Chest x-ray usually shows single or multiple well-defined infiltrates. The chest x-ray, which showed a cavitary lesion in our patient, was done as a preoperative evaluation before removal of the subcutaneous nodule. Pulmonary cavitation is an infrequent finding in cryptococcosis. Pleural effusion, diffuse interstitial pattern, and hilar adenopathy are also uncommon. Calcification is not a feature of cryptococcosis.

Cutaneous cryptococcosis: It usually suggests disseminated infection. In the early stage, skin lesions are small painless papules or nodules as in this patient. Later, they enlarge, soften centrally, and ulcerate.

Osseous cryptococcosis: Cryptococcosis may rarely produce osteolytic lesions in the bone and then presents as cold abscesses.

Other manifestation of cryptococcosis mentioned in Table 7-2 are rare.

Differential Diagnosis (Table 7-6)

Various conditions need to be differentiated from cryptococcosis, depending on the presenting feature as indicated in Table 7-6.

Diagnosis (Table 7-7)

Diagnosis of cryptococcosis requires a high degree of suspicion. All patients with predisposing conditions should have a regular follow-up and be educated to report any prolonged or unusual illness and any clinical feature suggesting infection should be thoroughly investigated. The physician looking after this group of patients should have a low threshold for lumbar puncture for headache.

Various measures for the diagnosis of cryptococcosis are listed in Table 7-5.

Treatment

Amphotericin with or without flucytosine has been the treatment of choice in all patients with cryptococcosis [5, 6]. However, several recent trials have suggested that fluconazole is very effective and can be used

Table 7-6. Differential Diagnosis of Cryptococcosis

Meningoencephalitis
  Tuberculosis
  Viral meningitis
  Histoplasmosis
  Coccidioidomycosis
  Candidiasis
  Sarcoidosis
  Neoplasm

Pulmonary cryptococcosis
  Tuberculosis
  Neoplasm
  Other fungal infections

Cutaneous cryptococcosis
  Comedo
  Basal cell carcinoma
  Sarcoidosis
  Molluscum contagiosum in AIDS patient

Osseous cryptococcosis
  Tuberculosis

Table 7-7.   Diagnosis of Cryptococcosis

Meningoencephalitis	
Cerebrospinal fluid (CSF)	
Glucose	<50 mg/dl in 67% of the patients
	<50% of serum glucose in 75% of the patients
Protein	50–300 mg/dl in 75% of the patients
Leukocytes	20–600/μl in 75% of the patients predominantly lymphocytes
India ink	Positive in 50% of the cases

Cryptococcal antigen Positive in serum and CSF in 90% of the patients
Positive CSF culture is the gold standard for diagnosis.
Urine is often positive for fungus.
Blood cultures are positive in 10–30% of the patients. They are positive more often in the AIDS patient.
Pulmonary cryptococcosis
  Serum test for cryptococcal antigen may be negative in 30% of the patients.
  Biopsy is the gold standard for diagnosis.
Cutaneous cryptococcosis
  Biopsy
Osseous cryptococcosis
  Biopsy

in all patients (except those with severe illness) with comparable results to standard therapy. Our patient was started on oral fluconazole. He remains well after more than 5 months of therapy. He remains well. There are no significant new skin lesions and the cavitary lung lesion is shrinking.

REFERENCES

1. Rubin RH, Infectious disease complications of renal transplantation. *Kidney Int* 1993;44:221–236.
2. Stamm AM, Dismukes WH. Cryptococcal neoformans infections. In Mandell GL, Douglas RG, Bennett JE, eds. *Principles and Practice of Infectious Diseases* (3rd ed), New York: Churchill Livingstone, 1990:1573–1577.
3. Bennett JE. Fungal infections. In Wilson JD, Braunwald E, Isselbacher KJ, Petersdorf RG, Martin JB, Fauci AS, Root RK, eds. *Harrison's Principles and Practice of Internal Medicine* (12th ed), edited by New York Mcgraw-Hill, 1991:743–744.

4. de Wytt CN et al. Cryptococcal meningitis: A review of 32 years' experience. *J Neurol Sci* 1982;53:283–292.

5. Conti DJ, Tolkoff-Rubin NE, Baker GP Jr, Doran M, Cosimi AB, Delmonico F, Auchincloss H J. Russell PS, Rubin RH. Successful treatment of invasive fungal infections with fluconazole in organ transplant recepients. *Transplantation* 1989;48:692–695.

6. Tolkoff-Rubin NE, Conti DJ, Doran M, Delvecchio A, Rubin RH. Fluconazole in the treatment of invasive candidal and cryptococcal infections in organ transplant recipients. *Pharmacotherapy* 1990;10(6, Pt. 3):159S–163S.

8

High-Grade Fever, Jaw Pain, and Abnormal Liver Function Tests after Wisdom Teeth Extraction in a Renal Transplant Patient

Mahendra V. Govani, Thomas L. McCurley, Robert C. MacDonell, Jr., and J. Harold Helderman

CASE PRESENTATION

History of Present Illness

A 28-year-old Caucasian man was admitted for high-grade fever and pain and swelling of the right jaw after ipsilateral wisdom teeth extraction 1 day before admission. He had received a 1B, 1DR matched cadaver kidney transplant 22 months earlier for end-stage renal disease (ESRD) from immune complex glomerulonephritis, probably membranoproliferative glomerulonephritis type III (MPGN III).

He had developed diabetes mellitus (DM) at age 2 in 1968. Signs of proliferative diabetic retinopathy appeared when he was 18 years old and his vision worsened quickly despite several laser treatments. Three years later, he was completely blind in the right eye and visual acuity was 20/400 in the left eye. In the same year, 4 weeks after an apparent varicella infection, he developed rapidly progressive renal failure for which a renal biopsy was performed at another hospital. It showed endocapillary and mesangial proliferation with widespread immune deposits predominantly in the subendothelial region; there was also evidence of mild diabetic glomerulopathy. The biopsy findings were thought to be consistent with lupus nephritis (WHO class IV). However, there were no extrarenal manifestations of systemic lupus erythematosus, antinuclear antibody (ANA) was negative, complement levels were normal, and there were no reticular arrays in the endothelial cell cytoplasm. The diagnosis of MPGN III was thought to be more likely. It was concluded that he had an immune complex glomerulonephritis of uncertain etiology and a trial was justified with high-dose glucocorticoids that were initiated along with hemodialysis. His renal function improved slowly and hemodialysis was discontinued after 6 months. Later that year, enucleation of the right eye and vitrectomy with laser photocoagulation were performed on the left eye.

During the next 4 years, diabetic retinopathy was his major problem and he had several more laser treatments on the left eye. He also had cataract extraction with lens implantation in the left eye approximately 3 years before admission. Six months later, the diagnosis of generalized sensorimotor polyneuropathy was made. His renal function gradually deteriorated during this time and he was put on the waiting list for cadaver kidney transplant 26 months before admission. Access was reconstructed on his left forearm in preparation for hemodialysis.

After 4 months on the waiting list, he received a 1B, 1DR matched cadaver kidney. The graft functioned immediately and his creatinine dropped to 1.4 from 5.9 after 3 days. He received rabbit antithymocyte serum (RATS), azathioprine, and glucocorticoids for induction. On the third posttransplant day, cyclosporine was started and RATS was stopped on the 12th day, when stable levels of cyclosporine were achieved. His stay in the hospital was unremarkable except for difficult control of DM because of high doses of glucocorticoids.

After 13 months of decent transplant function, he developed dysuria and frequency of urine with 4+ hematuria. Cystoscopy revealed an inflamed bladder, biopsy of which showed adenovirus infection of the bladder. The rest of the evaluation was normal and renal function was stable. His symptoms improved after a few days and hematuria resolved.

Two months later, hematuria reappeared with 2+ proteinuria. On urine microscopic examination, there were a few hyaline and fine granular casts. A 24-h urine protein excretion was 2.3 g, serum creatinine was stable at 1.7 mg/dl, ultrasound examination of the graft was normal, and I-125 iothalamate clearance was 73.5 ml/min/1.73 m². Transplant biopsy, performed 5 months later (approximately 6 weeks before admission) because of persistent hematuria and proteinuria, showed immune complex glomerulonephritis with widespread immune deposits. Again, there were no systemic manifestations of SLE; ANA was negative and complement levels were normal. It was thought that he had a recurrence of the original glomerular disease in the allograft and the decision was made to follow him closely in the outpatient clinic.

Three weeks before admission, he was asymptomatic with normal physical examination. Serum creatinine was 1.9 mg/dl, BUN was 29 mg/dl, and blood sugar was 173 mg/dl. Serum electrolytes, proteins, calcium, phosphorus, alkaline phosphatase, bilirubin, SGOT, LDH, and CBC were normal.

One day prior to admission, he had two wisdom teeth extracted on the right side without any immediate complications. He received prophylactic amoxycillin in appropriate doses before and after the dental procedure. On the day of admission, he complained of high fever with chills, and pain and swelling of the right jaw. He was not able to eat any solids but had no problems in keeping down liquids and his medications. There was no history of headache, cough, chest pain, dyspnea, abdominal pain, diarrhea, dysuria, or frequency of urine. He was on prednisone 5 mg bid, azathioprine 50 mg q hs, cyclosporine 150 mg bid, nifedipine XL 30 mg bid, clonidine 0.2 mg bid, sulfisoxazole 500 mg bid, and pentazocine PRN.

The patient consumed alcohol usually in moderation, but sometimes, he went on drinking binges. He had never smoked and there was no history suggestive of drug abuse or homosexual behavior. He lived with his mother, who was separated from his father. There was no family history of diabetes mellitus, SLE, hypertension, or renal disorder.

Physical Examination

Vital signs: Temperature 102.7°F, BP 184/106 mm Hg, pulse 137/min, and regular, RR 22/min.

The patient looked unwell, but he was not in any acute distress. There were no skin lesions. His right eye was prosthetic, and visual acuity of the left eye was poor with partial cataract. Left fundus examination revealed scarring from laser photocoagulation with normal optic disc. There was tender but nonfluctuant swelling on the right side of the face. The oral cavity was normal except for two missing wisdom teeth on the right side. The neck was supple; jugular venous pressure was not raised and there was no lymphadenopathy. Examination of heart and lungs was unremarkable. The abdomen was mildly distended without any tenderness. The renal allograft was nontender and there was no bruit. Bowel sounds were normal. Examination of the central nervous system was normal. Extremities were normal and there was no peripheral edema.

Laboratory Data

Urinalysis showed 4+ sugar, 2+ albumin, moderate amount of blood, and specific gravity of 1.024; there were 0–1 WBCs, 8–14 RBCs, 0–1 hyaline cast, and 0–1 coarse granular cast per high power field. Laboratory values are presented in Table 8-1, Electrocardiogram (EKG) revealed sinus tachycardia.

Radiologic Studies

Chest x-ray showed old granulomatous disease; there was no evidence of pulmonary edema, pleural effusion, or pulmonary infiltrates; cardiomediastinal silhouette and pulmonary vasculature were normal. X-ray of the abdomen revealed mild distension of stomach, small and large bowel in a uniform pattern suggesting mild ileus. Computed tomographic (CT) scan of the maxillofacial region demonstrated opacification of the right maxillary sinus suggestive of infection.

EARLY HOSPITAL COURSE

The patient was started on intravenous normal saline and sliding scale insulin. Blood cultures were taken and intravenous amoxycillin–sul-

Table 8-1. Laboratory Values on Admission

Hemoglobin	14G/dl
Hematocrit	40%
WBC	7.6×10^3 μl
Differential	
Neutrophils	77%
Lymphocytes	15%
Monocytes	4%
Eosinophils	2%
Metamyelocytes	2%
Platelets	154×10^3 μl
PT	15 s (INR 1.7)
PTT	25 s

NA 123 mEq/L, K 6 mEq/L, Cl 82 mEq/L, CO_2 19 mEq/L, glucose 612 mg/dl

BUN 68 mg/dl, creatinine 2.6 mg/dl

Ca 7.8 mg/dl, P 4.7 mg/dl, alkaline phosphatase 283 U/L

Total protein 5.2 g/dl, albumin 2.8 g/dl

Bilirubin 1.5 mg/dl, SGOT 65 U/L, LDH 1924 U/L

Uric acid 9.2 mg/dl

Triglycerides 327 mg/dl, cholesterol 141 mg/dl

Cyclosporine level 198 ng/ml

bactam was instituted. On the second hospital day, the temperature spiked to 104°F; hematocrit was 35, WBC count was $7.8 \times 10^3/\mu l$, and platelet count dropped to $57 \times 10^3/\mu l$; INR was 2.3, fibrinogen was 500 mg/dl, and fibrin split products titer was 1:32. Sulfisoxazole and azathioprine were discontinued, and intravenous aztreonam was added. On the fourth hospital day, his antibiotics were changed to vancomycin and piperacillin. Blood cultures were negative. Test for cytomegalovirus (CMV) antigen and CMV cultures were negative.

On the fifth day of admission, his abdominal distension got worse and he developed shortness of breath. He also had vague generalized abdominal pain which he had off and on since admission. Arterial blood pH was 7.41; pO_2 was 41 and pCO_2 was 31 mm of Hg at FIO_2 of 0.4; bicarbonate was 19 mmol/L. FIO_2 was increased to 0.5 and the patient's oxygenation was satisfactory. A nasogastric tube was introduced and his abdominal pain and distension improved. His antibiotic regimen was changed to vancomycin, ceftazidime, and metronidazole. The results of hematologic and blood chemical studies are listed in Table 8-2. Chest x-ray showed decreased lung volumes with bibasilar infiltrates and subsegmental atelectasis. Plain x-ray of the abdomen demonstrated worsening distension of the small and large bowel in a uniform pattern;

Table 8-2.   Laboratory Values on the Fifth Day of Admission

Hemoglobin	8.8 G/dl
Hematocrit	25%
WBC	$5.7 \times 10^3/\mu l$
Differential	
Neutrophils	64%
Lymphocytes	18%
Monocytes	11%
Eosinophils	2%
Metamyelocytes	2%
Atypical Lymphocytes	3%
Platelets	$42 \times 10^3/\mu l$
PT	17 s (INR 2.0)
PTT	29 s
Na 133 mEq/L, K 4.5 mEq/L, Cl 103 mEq/L, CO_2 14 mEq/L, glucose 88 mg/dl	
BUN 76 mg/dl, creatinine 2.6 mg/dl	
Total protein 5.8 g/dl, albumin 3.0 g/dl	
Bilirubin 1.6 mg/dl, SGOT 56 U/l, LDH 1421 U/L, alkaline phosphatase 272 U/L	
Lactic acid 1.2 mEq/L	

there was no free air suggesting perforation. Echocardiogram showed normal left ventricular function; there were no vegetations. Ventilation–perfusion scan disclosed matched defects in the lingular segment of the left upper lobe and in the superior segment of the right upper lobe, suggesting a low probability of pulmonary embolism. Ultrasound of the abdomen revealed a rounded, 3-cm lesion of mixed echogenicity in the posterior segment of the right lobe of the liver; the gallbladder was distended with echogenic material and the wall was slightly thickened, suggesting acalculus cholecystitis; a small amount of ascites was seen; there was no evidence of biliary obstruction; and there was a small lesion of mixed echogenicity in the inferior pole of the allograft. CT scan of the abdomen (Fig. 8-1) confirmed the lesions in the right lobe of the liver and in the allograft seen on ultrasound and it also showed another small lesion of low density in the anterior segment of the right lobe of the liver. HIDA scan was negative for cholecystitis. Ultrasound-guided liver biopsy was performed.

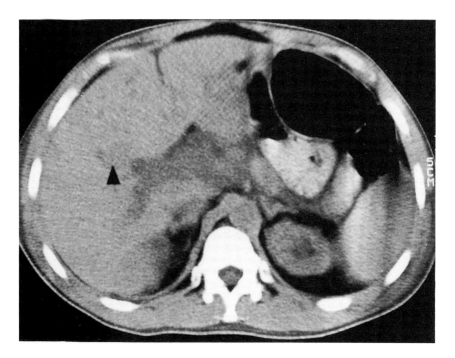

Figure 8-1. CT scan of the abdomen on the fifth day of admission revealing a low density lesion in the right lobe of the liver.

PATHOLOGY REPORTS

Fine-needle aspirate of the hepatic mass (Fig. 8-2) showed uniform population of noncohesive tumor cells with dispersed chromatin, 1–3 nucleoli, and basophillic vacuolated cytoplasm; mitotic figures were frequent. Immunologic typing studies by flow cytometry revealed B cell markers (CD19, CD20, CD10) with monotypic IgM kappa on the surface of the neoplastic cells. T cell markers were negative by indirect immunofluorescence.

Bone marrow biopsy was done to confirm the diagnosis of posttrans-

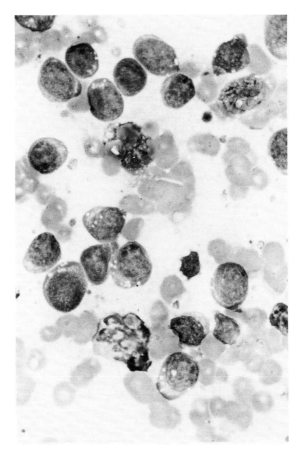

Figure 8-2. Fine-needle aspirate of the hepatic lesion showing neoplastic cells with scanty vacuolated dark cytoplasm (Wright stain ×1000)

plantation lymphoproliferative disorder (PTLD) and to stage the disease. The biopsy (Fig. 8-3) showed foci of marrow replacement by small transformed cells with moderate variation in size and shape. A morphological diagnosis of malignant lymphoma, small noncleaved cell (non-Burkitt's) type, was made. Cytogenetic studies showed a 46XY karyotype with a possible small 14q11 deletion.

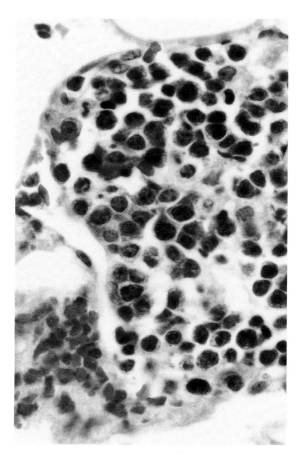

Figure 8-3. Bone marrow examination revealing replacement of the marrow by the neoplatic cells with moderate variation in size and shape; the nuclear diameter of the tumor cells is approximately that of the endothelial cell at the 9 o'clock position (periodic acid–Schiff ×630).

DIAGNOSIS

The diagnosis were posttransplantation lymphoproliferative disorder; monoclonal, rapidly progressive variety.

LATE HOSPITAL COURSE

The diagnosis and prognosis were discussed in detail with the patient, his mother, and his primary nephrologist. The dose of cyclosporine was reduced; acyclovir, gammaglobulin, and interferon alfa were started. Epstein-Barr virus (EBV) serology showed that the patient was EBV-negative 2 months earlier and was now strongly positive. CT scan of the head showed mild diffuse loss of brain substance with no paren-chymal abnormalities. The patient's condition continued to deteriorate; cyclosporine was tapered further and stopped. His graft function wors-ened and he was started on hemodialysis. CT scan of the abdomen (Fig. 8-4), performed several days later, revealed increased number and size of the lesions in the liver; there was also a moderate amount of ascites. Chemotherapy and prognosis were discussed in detail and the decision was made against chemotherapy. His condition worsened over the next few days and he died. The family did not agree to a postmortem ex-amination.

DISCUSSION

Posttransplantation lymphoproliferative disorder (PTLD), which is vir-tually always associated with Epstein-Barr virus (EBV), is an uncommon but potentially life-threatening complication of transplantation. It is a polyclonal or monoclonal neoplastic disorder of B cells, transformed and immortalized by EBV [1, 2].

PTLD was first reported in 1968. The incidence varies depending on the degree of immunosuppression associated with various organ transplants. The overall incidence is 1% in renal, 1.8% in heart, 2.2% in liver, and 4.6% in heart–lung transplant recipients. An incidence of greater than 20% has been reported in the recipients of T-cell-depleted bone marrow. It is more common in EBV-negative recipients and, therefore, in children who are more likely to be seronegative at the time of transplantation. However, considering the ubiquitous nature of EBV infection (prevalence more than 95% in the adult population of the

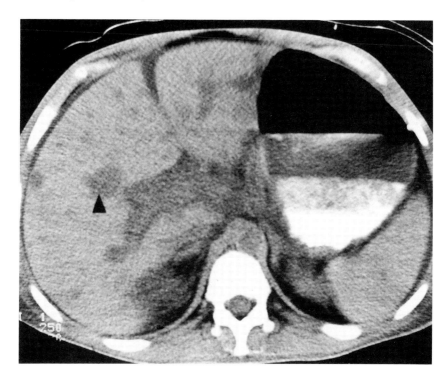

Figure 8-4. CT scan of the abdomen on the 19th day of admission demonstrating increased size of the lesion seen on the previous CT scan; several other low-density lesions are also seen.

Western Hemisphere) and the larger adult transplant recipient population, most cases of PTLD are reported in seropositive individuals.

Etiopathogenesis

The imbalance of host–EBV interactions is thought to be an important factor in the development of PTLD [3].

The portal of entry for EBV is usually the pharynx; however, it has been shown that it can be transmitted by organ transplantation. Infection is usually asymptomatic during early childhood and causes infectious mononucleosis frequently during adolescence or early adulthood. The virus replicates in pharyngeal epithelial cells and invades B lymphocytes through C3d receptors (also known as CR2 or CD21). The invaded B cells are immortalized and comprise up to 10% of total B lymphocytes in the peripheral circulation during active infection. MHC class I restricted EBV-specific cytotoxic T cells are the main defense against these immortalized B cells. These cytotoxic T cells recognize EBV+ B cells by EBV-specific peptides presented by class I MHC molecules on their surface, attack, and lyse them. For ill-defined reasons, EBV is never fully eradicated but enters into an unstable latent phase following acute infection.

During this latent phase, the virus continues to replicate in pharyngeal epithelial cells, and at any time, 20% of the seropositive individuals shed virus in pharyngeal secretions. EBV+ B cell pool size is thought to be <2 per million of circulating B lymphocytes and <1 per 10 million peripheral blood mononuclear cells in normal seropositive individuals. EBV-specific T cells continue to control the population of these EBV+ B cells. Replication of the virus in the pharynx can be inhibited by acyclovir or gancyclovir; however, these agents do not have any effect on EBV-transformed B cells.

Frequency of EBV isolation in the pharyngeal secretions is about 30% in the transplant EBV-seropositive population during stable immunosuppression and it rises to more than 70% during the treatment with antilymphocyte antibodies (especially monoclonal). PTLD is more likely to develop in transplant recipients with higher amount of replication and, therefore, shedding of the virus. Cyclosporine has been shown to impair the function of EBV-specific T cells. Other immunosuppressive agents, like azathioprine and glucocorticoids, also impair T-cell function to a lesser extent.

It has been shown recently that EBV+ B-cell pool size expands frequently 100–1000-fold after transplantation; however, most patients do not develop PTLD, suggesting that there is adequate and effective protection by EBV-specific T cells.

In some immunosuppressed patients, EBV-specific T-cell surveillance may not be adequate and EBV+ B-cell pool size grows unchecked leading to PTLD. It is also possible that some genetic mutation in EBV+ B cells leads them to divide faster, and this rapidly dividing pool of cells overwhelms immune surveillance. In some patients with PTLD, both of these mechanisms may be applicable.

Clinical Features

PTLD is less common and usually appears more than 2 years after transplantation in patients on azathioprine-based immunosuppression [4]. Since the introduction of cyclosporine and the wider use of antilymphocyte antibodies (especially monoclonal antibodies), PTLD has become more frequent and it usually presents within a few months after transplantation [5].

Depending on the clonality, presenting features, and course of the illness, PTLD may be divided in four ill-defined groups:

1. **Polyclonal, mononucleosis-like syndrome**. Usually benign. Large oropharyngeal lymphoid tissue may cause upper respiratory tract obstruction. Reducing immunosuppression usually helps.
2. **Polyclonal, rapidly progressive, fulminant diffuse PTLD**. Severe host defect. This syndrome resembles infectious mononucleosis in patients with X-linked lymphoproliferative syndrome. Death is common [6].
3. **Polyclonal and/or monoclonal, single or multiple lesions**. Most common variety of PTLD. It more frequently involves extranodal sites like brain, intestine, liver, lung, and allograft than typical lymphoma. It responds completely or partially to reducing the dose of immunosuppression.
4. **Monoclonal, rapidly progressive PTLD**. This variety of PTLD progresses very quickly despite immunomodulation [7].

Unfortunately, there are no definite criteria to help decide which group a patient belongs at presentation. Polyclonal and monoclonal disease may coexist. Cases of transformation from polyclonal to monoclonal variety have been reported. Also, cases initially thought to be monoclonal were demonstrated to be polyclonal on further morphological studies. Central nervous system (CNS) involvement is more common and the disease is more likely to have poor prognosis in the patients who are on azathioprine-based immunosuppression.

Clinical features are diverse and depend upon the organ involvement. They are presented in Table 8-4.

Our patient had PTLD involving several organ systems. The process was definitely demonstrated in the liver and the bone marrow. His abdominal distension was probably due to involvement of the bowel. A lesion seen in the allograft on the ultrasound and the CT scan of the abdomen might have been a result of the neoplastic process or the biopsy performed 6 weeks before admission. The clinical features and the chest x-ray findings suggestive of pulmonary pathology can be explained either by tumor invasion of the lungs or secondary infection.

Diagnosis

Diagnosis of PTLD requires a high degree of vigilance because of several reasons:

1. It is uncommon.
2. Undiagnosed and untreated, in time PTLD has a very high mortality.

3. It has a myriad of presentations (Table 8-3).
4. Each presenting feature has a large differential diagnosis.
5. PTLD is among the least common group of conditions in the differential diagnosis for any of the presenting features.

It cannot be overemphasized that any suspicious focal lesion should be biopsied in a transplant patient.

It may be difficult to differentiate allograft rejection from PTLD even after biopsy. Mononuclear cellular infiltration in the allograft may be interpreted as acute rejection and may get treated with increased immunosuppression leading to disastrous consequences. Therefore, whenever in doubt, cells of the mononuclear cellular infiltrate in the allograft should be characterized further.

Once the diagnosis is established, clonality may be determined by studies like surface immunoglobulin typing, gene rearrangement, or EBV genome termini structure [7, 8].

Our patient was asymptomatic 3 weeks before admission and his liver function tests were normal. Initially, it was thought that the patient had a periodontal abscess because of high-grade fever and jaw swelling with pain on the right side following wisdom teeth extraction on the same side. However, clinical signs were soft for periodontal abscess and it was difficult to explain abnormal liver function tests and mild paralytic ileus on that basis. Search for an intraabdominal process was continued and ultrasound-guided biopsy was performed, once a lesion was demonstrated in the liver. The diagnosis was established within a week of admission.

Table 8-3. Clinical Presentations of PTLD

Mononucleosis-like syndrome—mild variety
Mononucleosis-like syndrome—fulminant variety similar to one seen in the patients with X-linked lymphoproliferative syndrome
Tonsillar enlargement
Allograft dysfunction
Fever of unknown origin
Liver dysfunction
Focal gastrointestinal disease usually presenting as perforation, obstruction, or bleeding
Focal CNS disease
Focal pulmonary disease
Lymphadenopathy (uncommon)
Systemic inflammatory response syndrome (SIRS)

Management

Reduction or cessation of immunosuppression, especially cyclo-sporine, is the mainstay of treatment for PTLD [8]. This maneuver improves the effectiveness of EBV-specific cytotoxic T cells, which kill EBV-immortalized B cells. The response rate is good in patients with polyclonal, localized disease. Overall response rate is approximately 40%. Patients with CNS disease and/or monoclonal, rapidly progressive disease respond poorly. Acute graft rejection may develop and the graft may fail; however, the incidence of graft failure is not high. Once PTLD is eliminated, retransplantation can be done in the renal transplant recipients without much concern about recurrence of PTLD.

Antiviral agents, like acyclovir and gancyclovir, are effective against the replicating virus but not against the latent virus which is found in EBV-immortalized B cells. However, cases with successful outcome are reported when these agents were used and there are recent reports suggesting the presence of replicating virus in some of the PTLD cell lines. Further studies are needed before definite recommendations can be made about their use.

Interferon α and γ globulin have been shown to be effective in a small series of patients. However, interferon α can induce or exacerbate acute rejection.

Results of chemotherapy and radiotherapy are generally poor except occasional anecdotal reports of success.

Polyclonal PTLD without CNS involvement may go into remission with anti-B-cell monoclonal antibodies. However, further studies are necessary.

Papadopoulos et al. [11] recently used donor-derived cytotoxic T cells to treat monoclonal and polyclonal PTLD in patients who received T-cell-depleted bone marrow transplant. The treatment was highly effective. The treatment of PTLD in solid organ transplantation can be studied with a similar strategy where HLA matched EBV-specific cytotoxic T cells can be infused into the patient after they are separated and expanded in vitro [10, 11].

Surgical treatment may be necessary in the event of upper respiratory obstruction from enlarged lymphoid tissue in the pharynx or bowel perforation.

A severe combined immunodeficiency (SCID) mouse model has been developed for PTLD. Various therapeutic approaches can be tried on this model before human studies. Recently, it was shown that soluble CR2 prevented the development of PTLD in SCID mice.

Although research continues to determine effective treatment of

PTLD, the goal should be prevention. An ideal immunosuppressive regimen is one that prevents rejection and has minimal risk of infection. The transplant community continues to look for such a regimen. Meanwhile, all organ recipients and donors should be tested for EBV serology. EBV-negative individuals may receive lower doses of immunosuppression and treatment with monoclonal antibodies can be avoided altogether. EBV vaccine is being developed [12]. If it works, this will be a major advance in the prevention of PTLD and other EBV-associated illnesses.

Reduction and cessation of immunosuppression did not halt the progression of the disease in our patient. His graft loss was thought to be from acute rejection due to cessation of immunosuppression and probably treatment with interferon α. It is difficult to say whether he would have responded to monoclonal antibodies and/or chemotherapy or not. However, considering that his PTLD was the monoclonal, rapidly progressive variety involving several systems, this would have been unlikely.

ACKNOWLEDGMENTS

We are grateful to J. Stephen Dummer, M.D., Associate Professor of Medicine and Surgery at Vanderbilt University Medical Center, Nashville, Tennessee, for helpful comments.

REFERENCES

1. Liebowitz D, Kieff E. Epstein-Barr virus. In: Roizman B, Whitley RJ, Lopez C, eds. *The Human Herpesviruses.* New York: Raven Press, 1993:107–172.
2. Nalesnik MA. Lymphoproliferative disease in organ transplant recipients. *Springer Semin Immunopathol* 1991;13:199–216.
3. Rubin RH. Infectious disease complications of renal transplantation. *Kidney Int* 1993;44:221–236.
4. Craig PE, Gulley ML, Banks PM. Posttransplantation lymphoproliferative disorders. *Am J Clin Pathol* 1993;99(3):265–276.
5. Alfrey EJ, Friedman AL, Grossman RA et al. A recent decrease in the time to development of monomorphous and polymorphous posttransplant lymphoproliferative disorder. *Transplantation* 1992;54(2):250–253.
6. Purtilo DT. X-linked lymphoproliferative disease (XLP) as a model of Epstein-Barr virus-induced immunopathology. *Springer Semin Immunopathol* 1991;13:181–197.
7. Jones C, Bleau B, Buskard N et al. Simultaneous development of dif-

fuse immunoblastic lymphoma in recipients of renal transplants from a single cadaver donor. Transmission of Epstein-Barr virus and triggering by OKT3. *Am J Kidney Dis* 1994;23(1):130–134.

8. Crompton CH, Cheung RK, Donjon C et al. Epstein-Barr virus surveillance after renal transplantation. *Transplantation* 1994;57(8):1182–1189.

9. Benkerrou M, Durandy A, Fischer A. Therapy for transplant-related lymphoproliferative diseases. *Hematol Oncol Clin North Am* 1993;7(2):467–475.

10. Fischer A, Blanche S, Le Bidois J et al. Anti-B-cell monoclonal antibodies in the treatment of severe B-cell lymphoproliferative syndrome following bone marrow and organ transplantation. *N Engl J Med* 1991;324:1451–1456.

11. Papadopoulos EB, Ladanyi M, Emanuel D et al. Infusions of donor leukocytes to treat Epstein-Barr virus-associated lymphoproliferative disorder after allogenic bone marrow transplantation. *N Engl J Med* 1994;330:1185–1191.

12. Pearson GR, Levine PH. Epstein-Barr virus vaccine: The time to proceed is now! In: Roizman B, Whitley RJ, Lopez C, eds. *The Human Herpesviruses*. New York: Raven Press, 1993:349–356.

9

Heart Transplantation After the Modified Fontan Repair

Jan Muirhead and William H. Frist

HISTORY OF PRESENT ILLNESS

An 18-year-old male born with tricuspid atresia and ventricular septal defect was admitted to Vanderbilt University Medical Center with worsening congestive heart failure. During this admission he was referred to the heart transplant program for consideration as a transplant candidate.

Previous procedures included a balloon septostomy at age 2 days, a left modified Blalock-Taussig shunt at age 18 months, a right-sided Glenn shunt at age 4 years, and a definitive Fontan repair with Bjork modification, utilizing a right atrium–to–right ventricular conduit, at age 8 years. His health had been stable since the Fontan procedure without major medical complications or hospitalizations. He had a history of exercise intolerance, precluding participation in sports, recurrent chest pain primarily with exertion, palpitations, and cyanosis that increased with exertion and improved at rest.

He was admitted to Vanderbilt University Medical Center in December 1991 with increasing chest pain, occurring sometimes at rest, and cyanosis. He was on no cardiac medications. A chest x-ray film showed normal heart size and pulmonary markings. The electrocardiogram revealed sinus rhythm with second-degree atrioventricular (AV) block (Mobitz type I) and a right bundle branch block. An echocardiogram demonstrated a large left ventricle with decreased function and a shortening fraction of 21%. Cardiac catheterization demonstrated right-to-left atrial shunt, atrial sinusoids to the right lung, normal pulmonary artery pressures, severely depressed left ventricular function, a patent Glenn shunt, and a narrowed conduit between the right atrium and right ventricle (10 mm Hg gradient). Therapeutic interventions included short-term dobutamine infusion to improve ventricular performance, captopril for afterload reduction, and mexilitene for treatment of ventricular arrhythmias. The patient required two subsequent admissions within 2 months for treatment of atrial flutter and eventual placement of a dual-chambered pacemaker for atrioventricular block and sinus node dysfunction.

At the time of transplant evaluation, the patient was in the intensive care unit receiving dobutamine infusion (10 mcg/kg/min) for a 6-day period. His respiratory status was stable with baseline oxygen saturations at approximately 85%. All transplant laboratory tests and procedures were obtained. A cardiac catheterization was performed to assess his current hemodynamic status with particular attention to his left pulmonary artery morphology, as this artery was not visualized on the previous catheterization. Hemodynamic findings are listed in Table 9-1. The pulmonary arteriogram demonstrated normal morphology of the left pulmonary artery without distal stenosis. The study confirmed end-stage left ventricular dysfunction with secondary pulmonary hypertension.

After a complete medical and psychosocial assessment, the patient was accepted as a heart transplant candidate. For approximately 5 weeks the patient waited at home for the transplant. However, the patient's condition deteriorated, with increasing cyanosis, shortness of breath, anorexia, and abdominal distention requiring rehospitalization in the intensive care unit. Oxygen therapy, dobutamine infusion, intravenous diuretics, and further afterload reduction with nitroglycerine paste were instituted. Five days later he underwent heart transplantation.

Table 9-1. Pretransplant Cardiac Catheterization Pressures

RA = $\overline{25}$ mm Hg
RV = $\overline{20}$ mm Hg
LPA = 27/20 mm Hg
RA–RV gradient = 5 mm Hg

Abbreviations: RA = right atrium; RV = right ventricle; LPA = left pulmonary artery; RA–RV = right atrium–to–right ventricle.

ORTHOTOPIC HEART TRANSPLANTATION AND POSTOPERATIVE COURSE

Dissection of the heart from surrounding tissue in the mediastinum was difficult due to the presence of adhesions. Figure 9-1 illustrates the configuration of the patient's heart at the time of transplantation. Figures 9-2 and 9-3 illustrate removal of the recipient heart with takedown of the Glenn shunt and completion of the donor heart implant, respectively. The operation was complicated by excessive bleeding from the right pulmonary artery anastomosis, requiring that the patient be placed

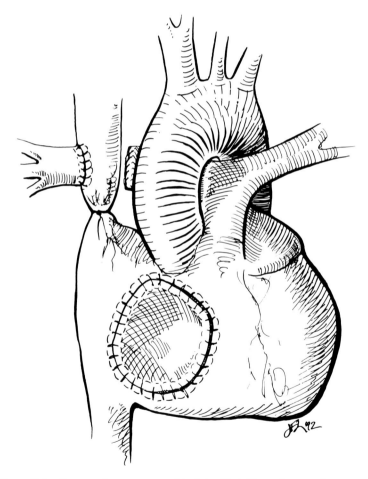

Figure 9-1. Pretransplant anatomy with right-sided Glenn shunt and Fontan repair with Dacron graft covering the Bjork modification.

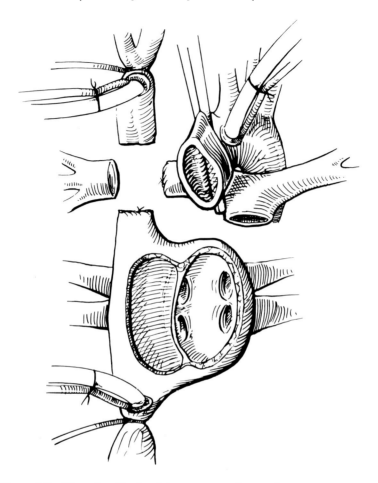

Figure 9-2. View of residual recipient anatomy after cardiectomy.

back on cardiopulmonary bypass and a Dacron graft be interposed between the donor and recipient right pulmonary arteries (Figure 9-3). Total donor ischemic time was 4 h 10 min. The immediate postoperative course was complicated by a coagulopathy necessitating multiple transfusions with fresh frozen plasma, platelets, and cryoprecipitate. The coagulopathy eventually resolved, but the patient returned to the operating room 18 h after the transplant was completed because of persistent bleeding. Reexploration of the mediastinum revealed diffuse bleeding from multiple surfaces with no evidence of tamponade. Postoperative inotropic support included isoproterenol (2.5 mcg/min) and

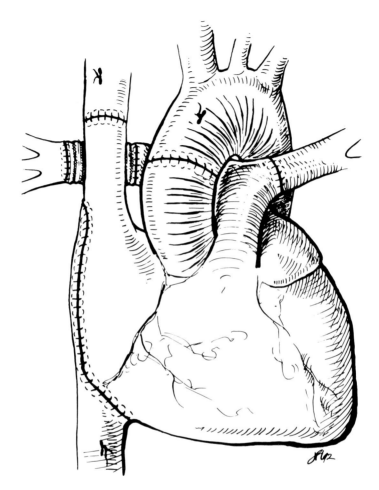

Figure 9-3. Posttransplant anatomy with right pulmonary artery interposition prosthetic material and separate anastomoses at superior vena cava, aorta, left pulmonary artery, and right atrium.

dopamine (5 mcg/kg/min) for 5 days. The patient was extubated on postoperative day 6 and transferred to the stepdown unit on day 8.

Preoperative immunosuppression included cyclosporine 400 mg p.o. and azathioprine 225 mg. Upon rewarming in the operating room, 500 mg of methylprednisolone was administered. An additional 125 mg of methylprednisolone was given for three doses, each 12 h apart, in the early postoperative period. Maintenance immunosuppression included cyclosporine p.o. to maintain trough levels of 250–300 ng/ml by the fluorescence polarized immune assay method the first 2 months, aza-thioprine 2 mg/kg/day, and prednisone beginning at 0.8 mg/kg/day and tapering by 0.1 mg/kg each week if the heart biopsy results remained negative. No induction therapy was given because of the need for reexploration of the mediastinum and concern about postoperative mediastinitis.

Rejection surveillance was accomplished with weekly transvenous right ventricular endomyocardial biopsies for approximately 8 weeks. The patient's first heart biopsy on day 10 showed mild rejection, grade IA. Because of intermittent mild rejection (grades IA and IB), prednisone dosage was tapered slowly during the first two postoperative months. The mild rejection episodes were treated with augmentation of cyclo-sporine and azathioprine dosages only.

Temporary atrial pacing was necessary for treatment of persistent bradycardia. Theodur (200 mg twice a day) was initiated to increase the sinus rate and allow discontinuation of the pacemaker. Right heart catheterization prior to discharge from the hospital demonstrated a pulmonary artery pressure of 40/10 mm Hg, a pulmonary vascular resistance (PVR) of 1.9 Wood units, and a cardiac output of 4.6 L/min. The patient was discharged to a local apartment on postoperative day 21.

OUTPATIENT FOLLOW-UP

The patient initially was seen in the clinic weekly for medical follow-up, gradually tapering to a once-a-month schedule. He attended a cardiac rehabilitation exercise program for approximately 6 weeks to build exercise tolerance and to improve muscle tone in preparation for the transition to home life. Cyclosporine levels have been maintained at 200–300 ng/ml. At 9 months posttransplant he has required no rehospitalizations for complications and is active at home, pursuing recreational and educational interests.

DISCUSSION

Complex congenital heart disease is a growing indication for heart transplantation in children, with approximately 44% of pediatric heart transplants performed in 1992 attributed to this diagnosis [1]. The evolution of appropriate recipient selection criteria and the development of improved operative techniques have made transplantation a reasonable alternative for children with end-stage congenital heart disease. The timing of transplantation depends on the natural history of the specific cardiac lesion and the relative risks and long-term benefits of conventional palliative treatment versus those of transplantation. Many children with congenital heart disease have undergone previous palliative and sometimes reparative procedures and present for transplantation once irreversible myocardial dysfunction has developed. This case study illustrates the difficulties associated with the evaluation of these patients for transplantation and the technical challenges involved in the perioperative and immediate postoperative periods.

Two factors that must be investigated thoroughly prior to transplantation in this population are pulmonary vascular resistance and pulmonary vessel anatomy. Some degree of pulmonary hypertension is common in patients with end-stage heart disease. A right heart catheterization must be performed to determine pulmonary pressures, PVR, and the degree to which increased pulmonary artery pressure and resistance will respond to vasodilator therapy. Generally accepted hemodynamic criteria after appropriate acute intervention includes a pulmonary artery systolic pressure usually less than 50 mm Hg, a PVR less than 3 Wood units (PVR index less than 6 Wood units), and a transpulmonary gradient less than 15 mm Hg [2, 3]. However, in many children with congenital heart disease, especially those with systemic-to-pulmonary artery shunts, accurate measurement of PVR is difficult because of unevenly distributed regional pulmonary blood flows and pressures. Moreover, determination of the degree of reversibility of pulmonary hypertension by the use of vasodilator agents is thought to be less predictable in patients with systemic-to-pulmonary artery shunts. Consequently, baseline pulmonary measurements may be the only data available when considering transplantation, thereby forcing the transplant team to estimate the likelihood that elevated PVR will be reversible after transplantation.

Distortion of the pulmonary artery anatomy by previous systemic-to-pulmonary artery shunts may present challenging technical problems during implantation of the donor heart leading to increased perioperative risk. The patient in this case study had undergone previous creation and subsequent takedown of a left Blalock-Taussig shunt, followed later by a right-sided classical Glenn shunt. The morphology of the pulmonary artery trunk and branches and the ability to reconstruct satisfactory pulmonary artery anatomy must be considered carefully when contemplating the transplant alternative for patients with complex congenital heart disease.

Reconstruction of the pulmonary arteries requires the use of additional lengths of donor aorta and pulmonary artery. During the transplant operation, the surgeon may have to improvise based on intraoperative anatomic findings [4]. An unexpected event during the case study patient's transplant operation was the need to use prosthetic material to relieve tension on the right pulmonary artery anastomosis by lengthening the right pulmonary artery.

During the immediate postoperative period, excessive bleeding can be a problem caused by tedious dissection of mediastinal scar tissue and a prolonged period of extracorporeal circulation with possible development of a coagulopathy. Intensive support with the infusion of blood products, close monitoring for the development of tamponade, and judicious timing of reoperation for persistent bleeding are crucial decisions in the successful management of these patients.

Patients with complex congenital heart disease assume an increased perioperative and immediate postoperative risk of mortality and morbidity related to correction of congenital abnormalities and necessary modification of the transplant technique that might extend the operative, extracorporeal circulation, and graft ischemic times [5]. This case study demonstrates that once beyond the immediate posttransplant period these patients obtain an improved level of functioning unrealized prior to transplantation.

REFERENCES

1. Kaye, M. The registry of the International Society for Heart and Lung Transplantation: ninth official report—1992. *J Heart Lung Transplant* 1992;11:599–606.
2. Addonizio LJ, Gersony WM, Robbins RC et al. Elevated pulmonary vascular resistance and cardiac transplantation. *Circulation* 1987;76(Suppl. V):V52–V55.
3. Fricker FJ, Trento A, Griffith BP. Pediatric cardiac transplantation. *Cardiovasc Clin* 1990;20:223–235.
4. Cooper MM, Fuzesi L, Addonizio LJ, Hsu DT, Smith CR, Rose EA. Pediatric heart transplantation after operations involving the pulmonary arteries. *J Thorac Cardiovasc Surg* 1991;102:386–395.
5. Chartrand C, Guerin R, Kangah M, Stanley P. Pediatric heart transplantation: Surgical considerations for congenital heart diseases. *J Heart Transplant* 1990;9:608–617.

10

Soluble Circulating Intercellular Adhesion Molecule-1 (cICAM-1) in the Serum of Heart Transplant Patients Serum as an Indicator of Rejection: Correlation to Biopsy and Rejection

Xiaoming Zhao and William H. Frist

AIM OF THE STUDY

The aim of this project is to study the correlation of circulating ICAM-1 in transplant patient sera and the rejection; therefore, providing a new, convenient means of diagnosing the rejection, monitoring the treatment, and the role of adhesion molecules in host immune response.

SIGNIFICANCE

Adhesion molecules may play very important roles in transplant rejection but studying the dynamics of adhesion molecules in transplant patients remains difficult. The measurement of the level of adhesion molecules in transplant patient serum may help to develop a new, no-invasive method to monitor rejection, treatment, and, most importantly, a unique means of studying the role of adhesion molecules in host immune response following allograft.

REVIEW

The adhesion interactions of cells with other cells and with an extracellular matrix have a central role in the functions of the immune system [1]. Three families of cell-surface adhesion molecules regulate the migration of lymphocytes and interactions of activated cells during immune responses. They are the immunoglobulin superfamily, which includes an intercellular cell adhesion molecule (ICAM-1) and vascular cell adhesion molecule (VCAM-1); the integrin family, which is important in dynamic regulation of adhesion and migration, and the selectins, which are prominent in the lymphocyte and neutrophil interaction with vascular endothelium.

ICAM-1, a member of an immunoglobulin family with a five-domain structure (an 80–110-kD glycoprotein) has recently been characterized as one of the ligands to lymphocyte function associated antigen-1 (LFA-1) molecule [2, 3]. ICAM-1 can be expressed on a wide variety of cells, and its induction in inflammation is an important means of regulating LFA-1/ICAM-1 interactions [4, 5] and thereby presumably inflammatory responses.

ICAM-1 may play an important role in transplant rejection. γ-interferon, interleukin-1, and tumor necrosis factor can cause strong induction of ICAM-1 in a wide variety of tissues and greatly increase binding of lymphocyte and monocyte though their cell surface LFA-1 [4–7]. Endothelial cells that are exposed to cytokines result in enhanced expression and receptor activity of adhesion molecules, including ICAM-1 [8].

The prevalence of ICAM-1 and VCAM-1 expression has been found in the cardiac allograft biopsy. Some studies have reported that the increasing expression of ICAM-1 and VCAM-1 correlated with the incidence of allograft rejection [9]. Anti-ICAM-1 (R6.5) has been demonstrated to prolong graft survival in animal models [10]. It has also showed a reversing effect on the ongoing rejection [11]. In in vitro studies, monoclonal antibodies against human ICAM-1 and VCAM-1 have been shown to inhibit leukocyte adhesion to endothelial cells, granulocyte migration through endothelium, mitogen and Ag-induced lymphocyte proliferation, and mixed lymphocyte reaction [12–16].

Although it is generally believed that ICAM-1 and VCAM-1 may play an important role in transplant rejection, the study of ICAM-1 and

VCAM-1 in transplant patients in vivo remains difficulty. Some researchers reported the existence of a soluble form of ICAM-1 in human serum [17]. The soluble circulating ICAM-1 level increased in a variety of diseases [2, 18]. It would be expected that the soluble circulating ICAM-1 may increase due to the transplant rejection. Measuring the soluble circulating ICAM-1 level in the heart transplant patients will help to develop an new, noninvasive method to monitor the rejection, treatment, and most importantly, a unique means of studying the role of adhesion molecules in immune responses following allograft.

METHODS AND MATERIAL

Patients

The patients will come from heart transplant patients performed at the Vanderbilt Transplant Center. Approval by the committee and consent from the patient will be obtained. The blood will be collected at the same time as the routine test at monthly intervals for the first 3 months, and at 3-month intervals thereafter. Pretransplant blood will be stored in order to compare with posttransplant blood. Healthy human blood and "normal open heart" patients' (CABG) blood will serve as controls.

Monoclonal Antibodies

Mouse mAb R6.5 directed against domains 1 and 2 of ICAM-1 and mAb CL203.4 directed against domain 4 of ICAM will be used to detect circulating ICAM using enzyme-linked immunosorbent assay (ELISA) method.

Two-site ELISA for cICAM-1 and sICAM-1

mAb CL203.4 (10 µg/ml in DPBS) will be added to 96-well flat-bottom E.L.A. Microtiter plates at 50 µl/well at room temperature for 1 h. Wells will be washed three times with DPBS and then blocked with 200 µl of 2% BSA-DPBS for 1 h at 37 °C. Wells will be flicked empty and a titration of sICAM-1 standards (twofold serial dilutions 8–1024 ng/ml) and serum samples (diluted in 1% BSA-DPBS) will be added (50 µl/well) in triplicate for 1 h at 37 °C. After being washed with DPBS, the wells will be incubated with biotinylated anti-ICAM-1 mAb (R6.5) at 2 µg/ml (50 µl/well) for 30 min at 37 °C and, consequently, with an aliquot of 50 µl/well of horseradish peroxidase streptavidin (1:4000) for 30 min at 37 °C. Wells will be washed with DPBS and once with ABTS substrate buffer. ABTS substrate buffer will be then added (50 μl/well) and the plates will be read on a Microtiter ELISA reader (410 nm). cICAM-1 concentrations will be calculated from a log-logit analysis curve generated from the sICAM-1 titration.

Cardiac Allograft Biopsy

Cardiac allograft biopsy is routinely performed at the Vanderbilt Transplant Center. The specimens used in this study will be snap-frozen in OCT compound. The sections will be stained by hematoxylin-eosin and monoclonal antibodies. Anti-ICAM-1 monoclonal antibody will be used for the immunohistology study.

Statistics

The comparison will be carried out between the patients with ongoing rejection and without rejection, pretransplant, and posttransplant by Wilcoxon rank sum test.

REFERENCES

1. Springer TA. Adhesion receptors of the immune system. *Nature* 1990;346:425–434.
2. Shijbo N, Imai K, Aoki S. Circulating intercellular adhesion molecules-1 (ICAM-1) antigen in sera of patients with idiopathic pulmonary fibrosis. *Clin Exp Immunol* 1992;89:58–62.
3. Marlin SD, Springer TA. Purified intercellular adhesion molecule-1 (ICAM-1) is a ligand for Lymphocyte Function- Associated Antigen-1 (LFA-1).
4. Kishimoto TK, Larson RS, Corbi AL. The leukocyte integrins. *Adv Immunol* 1989;46:149–182.
5. Dustin ML, Staunton DE, Springer TA. Supergene families meet in the immune system. *Immunol Today* 1988;9:213–215.
6. Springer TA, Dustin ML, Kishimoto TK. The lymphocyte function-associated LFA-1, CD2, and LFA-3 molecules: Cell adhesion receptors of the immune system. *Annu Rev Immunol* 1987;5:223–252.
7. Dustin ML, Springer TA. Lymphocyte function-associated antigen-1 (LFA-1) interaction with intercellular adhesion molecule-1 (ICAM-1) is one of at least three mechanism for lymphocyte adhesion to cultured endothelial cells. *J Cell Biol* 1988;107:321–331.
8. Suciu-foca N, Reed E, Marboe C. The role of anti-HLA antibodies in heart transplantation. *Transplantation* 1991;51:716–724.

9. Allen MD, McDonald TO, Carlos T. Endothelial adhesion molecules in heart transplantation. *J Heart Lung Transplant* 1992;11:58–63.

10. Cosimi AB, Conti D, Delmonico FL. In vivo effects of monoclonal antibody to ICAM-1 (CD54) in nonhuman primates with renal allografts. *J Immunol* 1990;144:4604–4612.

11. Wee LS, Cosimi AB, Preffer FI. Functional consequences of anti-ICAM-1 (CD54) in cynomolgus monkeys with renal allografts. *Transplant Proc* 1991;23:279–280.

12. Smith CW, Rothlein R, Hughes J. Recognition of an endothelial determinant for CD18-dependent neutrophil adherence and transendothelial migration. *J Clin Invest* 1988;82:1746.

13. Smith CW, Marlin SD, Rothlein R. Cooperative interactions of LFA-1 and Mac-1 with intercellular adhesion molecule-1 in facilitating adherence and transendothelial migration of human neutrophils in vitro. *J Clin Invest* 1989;83:2008.

14. Dougherty GJ, Murdoch JS, Hogg N. The function of human intercellular adhesion molecule-1 (ICAM) in the generation of an immune response. *Eur J Immunol* 1987;180:35.

15. Boyd AW, Wawryk SO, Burns GF. Intercellular adhesion molecule-1 (ICAM-1) has a central role in cell-cell contact-mediated immune mechanisms. *Proc Natl Acad Sci USA* 1988;85:3095.

16. Merluzzi VJ, Rothlein R, Wood C. Inhibition of human mixed lymphocyte reactions by monoclonal antibodies to intercellular adhesion molecule-1 (ICAM-1). In: Springer TA, ed. *Leukocyte Adhesion Molecules*. New York: Springer-Verlag, 244.

17. Rothlein R, Mainolfi EA, Czajkowski M. A form of circulating ICAM-1 in human serum. *J Immunol* 1991;147:3788–3793.

18. Tsujisaki M, Imai K, Hirata H. Detection of circulating intercellular adhesion molecule-1 antigen in malignant diseases. *Clin Exp Immunol* 1991;85:3–8.

11

Cardiac Allograft Vasculopathy: Correlation with Immunoglobulin-Secreting Cell Activity in Peripheral Blood

Xiaoming Zhao and William H. Frist

AIM OF THE STUDY

Chronic rejection is responsible primarily for late loss of allografted organ. Indeed, despite important improvements in immunosuppression and in overall recipient care, the rate of attrition after the years of transplants regardless of type has not improved [1, 2]. The etiology of the cardiac allograft vasculopathy remains obscure. This study is designed to determine the relationship of peripheral blood B lymphocyte activity in heart transplant patients to cardiac allograft vasculopathy using an in vitro method. These specific aims were established:

1. The relationship of immunoglobulin-secreting cell count to CAV using reverse hemolytic plaque assay.
2. The relationship of donor-specific B lymphocyte response to CAV using mixed lymphocyte culture and reverse hemolytic plaque assay
3. The correlation of peripheral blood B lymphocyte activity and anti-HLA antibodies generation in transplant patient.

SIGNIFICANCE

The study of relationship between B lymphocyte activity and the cardiac allograft vasculopathy in heart transplant patients will contribute to the understanding of the etiology of CAV, therefore to developing an effective treatment to prevent cardiac allograft vasculopathy, and finally improve the long-term results of organ transplant. It also helps to develop a new method to predict CAV and monitor the efficiency of the treatment.

REVIEW

Survival after heart transplantation has improved steadily over the past decade with 1-year mortality rates now less than 15% [3]. Despite a substantial improvement in early survival, long-term results have not been improved. The major cause is cardiac allograft vasculopathy (CAV). CAV is a diffused process and occurs in between 15% and 20% of patients per year [1, 2]. In patients surviving at least 3 years, the prevalence may be as high as 45% [1].

The pathogenic mechanisms responsible for the development of CAV are unknown. Most studies have found no correlation between the presence of traditional "risk factors" and the propensity to develop CAV. Hypercholesterolemia, the lack of anticoagulant/antiplatelet therapy, and multiple episodes of rejection have not been related to the high incidence of CAV [1, 2, 4, 5].

The etiology of CAV is not fully understood. In contrast to naturally occurring arteriosclerosis, CAV lesions are usually concentric and diffused rather than focal. The consistent finding of T-cells and macrophages [6, 7] in graft atherosclerotic lesions and the demonstration of immunoglobulin and complement deposition [8] in affected vessel walls suggest that those abnormalities occur on an immunological basis. In clinical heart transplantation, the effect of HLA and numbers of early rejection episodes have correlated with the development of later graft CAV [5].

The relationship of cytotoxic antibodies to endothelial injury and arteritis in rejection has long been documented. Humoral activity has been thought to be responsible for CAV, as immunoglobulin and complement deposits have been shown in area of intimal thickening [9]. The process can be produced histologically by intraarterial infusion of donor-specific antisera [10]. A correlation between the development of graft atherosclerosis and anti-HLA antibodies has been described in renal graft [11]. One study showed that the 4-year survival among antibody nonproducers was 90% and among antibody producers 50%. The incidence of graft CAV was considerably higher in the latter group [12].

Some studies have implicated B-cell antibodies in the development of CAV. The presence of cytotoxic B-cell antibodies associated with hyperlipidemia correlated closely with the incidence of myocardia infarction and sudden death [4]. It has been suggested that donor-specific cytotoxic antibody inflicts early injury on coronary endothelium; B-cell antibodies then bind to DR antigen on the endothelium, initiating complement fixation on antibody-dependent cytotoxicity.

Antibodies eluted from chronically rejecting allografts showed both antidonor specificities of different types as well as nonspecific HLA antibodies [13]. Similarly, eluted anti-B-cell antibodies from such grafts react against endothelial cells [14, 15]. Some non-HLA antibodies against minor histocompatible antigens may contribute to the development of CAV as well [16].

Although antibody-mediated chronic rejection may play a very important role in CAV, there is no convincing evidence to confirm the hypothesis. Since antibody generation is postulated to be more active in those patients who develop CAV, B lymphocyte activity would be expected to be higher as well. Weimer and colleges demonstrated that the activity of immunoglobulin-secreting cells was significantly higher in patients with an ongoing rejection than those without rejection [17, 18]. But, the relationship of B-cell activity to CAV has not been addressed before. The understanding of the etiology of CAV and deleterious CAV on long-functioning allografts make it an important subject for the investigation.

METHODS AND MATERIAL

Patient

The patients will come from heart transplant patients at the Vanderbilt Transplant Center. Approval by the ethic committee and consent from the patients will be obtained. The study will not have any harmful effect on the patients. The peripheral blood will be collected at the same time as the routine test at monthly intervals for the first 3 months, and at 3-month intervals thereafter. The blood will be sent for various B lymphocyte activity tests and anti-HLA antibody screens. Cardiac allograft vasculopathy will be diagnosed as standard criterium.

Preparation of Lymphocytes

Peripheral blood lymphocytes will be separated from heparinized blood by Ficoll-Hypaque gradient centrifugation. The cells will be washed three times with Hank's balanced salt solution for reverse hemolytic plaque assay and flow cytometry assay. The cells for mixed lymphocyte culture will be washed in completed medium (RMPI 1640 supplemented with 2 mM L-glutamine, 10 mM HEPES solution, 100 U/ml penicillin, 100 mg/ml streptomycin, and 20% human serum). B-lymphocyte-enriched population will be separated from PBL by the Rosetting method [19].

Mixed Lymphocyte Culture

Mixed lymphocyte culture will be used to measure recipient B-cells response to donor spleen cells and various mitogens. PBL (10^5 cells) from the heart recipient will be cultured with donor spleen cells (10^5 cells, irradiated by 3700 rads), pokeweed mitogen (PWM, Gibco), *staphylococus aureus* Cowan I (SAC I) or without mitogen in a total volume of 200 μl completed medium in 96-well round-bottom plates at 37°C in 95% air/5% CO_2. All cell cultures will be performed in duplicate. After a 6-day culture period, the cells will be washed and plated in a reverse hemolytic plaque assay. B-cell-enriched lymphocytes will be incubated with donor spleen cells (irradiated), PWN, SAC-I, or without mitogen. Supernatant from Con-A stimulated spleen cells will serve as a source of cytokines. Third-party human PBL or irrelevant organ donor spleen cells (irradiated) will be used as the stimulator in MLC for control. After a 5-day culture period, each well will be pulsed with 1 μCi tritiated thymidine for 18 h prior to harvesting. Radioactivity will be measured in a scintillation counter.

Reverse Hemolytic Plaque Assay

The protein A modification of hemolytic plaque assay will be used for detection of immunoglobulin-secreting cell count. Protein A will be coupled to sheep red blood cells (SRBC) by the $CrCl_3$ method. Rabbit antihuman IgG/IgA/IgM will be incubated at 56°C for 30 min and absorbed with packed SRBC 1:1 for 1 h at 4°C. Guinea pig complement will be absorbed with packed SRBC at a 1:5 ratio for 1 h at 4°C. One hundred microliters of PBL at a concentration of 10^6/ml, and 25 μl protein A-coupled SRBC will be added to 250 μl Seaplaque agarose, mixed, and plated on a petri dish covered with Seakem ME agarose. The preabsorbed rabbit antihuman IgG/IgA/IgM will be added for 1 h at 37°C in a 5% CO_2-humidified atmosphere. Further addition of preabsorbed GPC will be followed by a 1-h incubation under the same conditions. Plaque will be counted by dark-field microscopy. Results will be expressed as PFC/10^6 PBL.

Flow Cytometry Assay

Expression of surface markers of B lymphocytes will be measured by flow cytometry assay. PBL will be prepared as described above and washed in the Hank's medium with 2% heat-inactivated fetal bovine serum (FBS), adjusted to 2×10^7/ml in Hank's medium with 10% FBS and incubated at 37°C for 20 min to minimize nonspecific antibody binding. The cells will be incubated with CD19-PE and CD23, CD11a/CD18, CD49d/CD29, or anti-IgM monoclonal antibodies, then incubated with second antibody (goat against rabbit IgG conjugated with FITC). The cells will be washed once and fixed in FACS fixative and analyzed using a flow cytometer.

Statistics

The comparison will be carried out between the patients with clinical CAV and those without CAV using the Student's *t*-test and Wilcoxon rank sum test.

REFERENCES

1. Uretsky BF, Murali S, Reddy PS. Development of coronary artery disease in cardiac transplant patients receiving immunosuppressive therapy with cyclosporine and prednisone. *Circulation* 1987;76:827–33.
2. Billingham ME. Cardiac transplant atherosclerosis. *Transplant Proc* 1987;19(Suppl. 5):19–25.
3. Kriett JM, Kaye MP. *J Heart Lung Transplant* 1990;9:323–330.
4. Hess JL, Hastillo A, Mohanakumar T. Accelerated atherosclerosis in cardiac transplantation: Role of cytotoxic B-cell antibodies and hyperlipidemia. *Circulation* 1983;68(Suppl. 2):94–101.
5. Gao SZ, Schroeder JS, Alerman EL. Clinical and laboratory correlates of accelerated coronary artery disease in the cardiac transplant patient. *Circulation* 1987;76:56–61.
6. Hruban RH, Beschorner WE, Baumgartner WA. Accelerated arteriosclerosis in heart transplant recipients is associated with a T-lymphocyte-mediated endothelialitis. *Am J Pathol* 1990;137:871–882.
7. Usy CJ, Rose AG. Cardiac transplantation: Aspects of the pathology. *Pathol Annu* 1983;17:147.
8. Palmer DC, Tsai CC, Roodman ST. Heart graft arteriosclerosis. *Transplantation* 1985;39:385.
9. Mohanakumar T, Rhodes C, Mendes-Picon G. Renal allograft rejection associated with pre-sensitization to HLA-DR antigen. *Transplantation* 1981;31:93.

10. O'Connell TX, Mobray JF. Arterial intimal thickening produced by alloantibody and xenoantibody. *Transplantation* 1990;51:262.

11. Reemtsma K. Vascular immunoobliterative disease is a common cause of graft failure. *Transplant Proc* 1989;21:3706.

12. Rose EA, Smith CR, Petrossian GA. Humoral immune response after cardiac transplantation: Correlation with fatal rejection and atherosclerosis. *Surgery* 1983;106:203.

13. Busch GJ, Schamberg JF, Moretz RL. T and B cell patterns in irreversibly rejected human renal allograft: correlation of morphology with surface markets and cytotoxic capacity of the isolated lymphoid infiltrates. *Lab Invest* 1976;35:272.

14. Mohanakumar T, Waldrop TC, Phibbs M. Serological characterization of antibodies eluted from chronically rejected human renal allografts. *Transplantation* 1981;32:61.

15. Ende N, Orsi EV, Baturay NZ. Properties of cytotoxic kidney antibodies associated with human renal transplantation. *Am J Clin Pathol* 1979;71:543.

16. Hewitt CW, Black KS, Harmon JC. Partial tolerance in rat renal allograft recipients following multiple blood transfusions and concomitant cyclosporin. *Transplantation* 1990;49:194.

17. Weimer R, Daniel V, Pomer S. B lymphocyte response as an indicator of renal transplant rejection. I. Immunoglobulin-secreting cells in peripheral blood. *Transplantation* 1989;48:569–572.

18. Weimer R, Daniel V, Pomer S. B lymphocyte response as an indicator of acute renal transplant rejection. II. Pretransplant and posttransplant B cell responses of mitogen and donor cell-stimulated culture. *Transplantation* 1989;48:572–575.

19. Galili V, Schlesinger M. The formation of stable E rosettes after neuraminidase treatment of either human peripheral blood lymphocytes or sheep red blood cells. *J Immunol* 1974;112:1628–1634.

20. Gronowicz E, Coutinbo A, Melchers F. A plaque assay for all cells secreting Ig of a given type or class. *Eur J Immunol* 1976;6:588–590.

12

The Effects of RS-61443 on the Expression of Adhesion Molecules on T Lymphocyte, B Lymphocyte, and Endothelial Cells: Prevention of Atherosclerosis of the Transplanted Heart

Xiaoming Zhao and William H. Frist

AIM OF THE STUDY

RS-61443, the morpholinoethyl ester of mycophenoloc acid (MPA) is a potent immunosuppressant with a profile of activities distinct from those of cyclosporine and FK 506. The aim of this study is to determine the effects of RS-61443 on the expression of adhesion molecules using in vitro and in vivo methods. Four specific aims of our study were developed.

1. The effects of RS-61443 on the adhesion molecules expression on the T lymphocytes, B lymphocytes, and endothelial cells induced by various cytokines and mitogen using monoclonal antibodies and flow cytometry assay

2. The effects of RS-61443 on the proliferation of T and B lymphocytes stimulated by various cytokines and mitogen using mixed lymphocyte culture technique and the cytotoxic assay

3. The effects of RS-61443 on the prevention of atherosclerosis of post-transplant heart (in rat model)
4. The effects of RS-61443 on the prevention of sensitization to the antibody type immunosuppressants (ATG and OKT3)

SIGNIFICANCE

The understanding of the effects of RS-61443 on the lymphocytes and the effects on the prevention of atherosclerosis will contribute to the improvement of long-term results of organ transplantation. It also offers the possibility for further study about xenografts.

REVIEW

Survival after heart transplantation has improved steadily over the past decade with 1-year mortality rates now less than 15% [1]. Despite a substantial improvement in early survival, late death has not been significantly impacted. The major cause of late death and graft failure is due to cardiac allograft vasculopathy (CAV). The incidence of this vascularpathy is between 15% and 20% [2, 3] of patients per year, and in patients surviving at least 3 years the prevalence may be as high as 45% [2]. The pathogenic mechanisms responsible for the development of CAV are unknown. It is generally believed that the initial event leading to the development of chronic vascular rejection, like atherosclerosis, results from injury to endothelial cells mediated by humoral rejection [4, 5].

Advances in immunosuppression during the last decade have made it possible to control acute rejection. Further success depends on the development of agent that are capable of reversing or preventing chronic rejection. Current immunosuppressive agents such as cyclosporine and FK 506 affect mainly T cells. New immunosuppressants should have the capability of controlling antibody-mediated reaction in host as well; one such immunosuppressant could be RS-61443.

RS-61443, an ester prodrug of mycophenolin acid (MPA), is a allosteric inhibitor of inosine monophosphate dehydrogenase (IMPDH), the rate-controlling enzyme of the purine de novo synthesis of guanine nucleotide, and guanosine monophosphate synthetase [6]. Antigen-activated B and T lymphocytes are highly dependent on purine de novo synthesis [7], whereas most other cells are capable of utilizing a salvage pathway.

Changes in nucleotide pools due to IMPDH inhibition are well characterized and produce specific depletion of intracellular GTP and dGTP pools [8]. GTP is necessary for protein and nucleic acid synthesis as well as several enzymatic reaction [9]. GTP is also required for the efficient translation of external signals into the production of second messengers in the interaction of cytokines and B lymphocytes [10]. Depletion of the GTP pool would be expected to block the proliferation and differentiation of B and T lymphocytes. It is possible that RS-61443 could be used as a selected potent immunosuppressive agent to control cellular and antibody-mediated rejection.

One important activity of RS-61443 (MPA) is the inhibition of primary and secondary antibody responses. This is shown in cultures of polyclonally stimulated human lymphocytes and in secondary responses of human spleen cells to antigen [11, 12]. In these models, therapeutically attainable doses of MPA or RS-61443 are strongly suppressive, whereas those of cyclosporine or FK 506 are not. In view of the potential role of antibodies in the proliferative vasculopathy associated with chronic rejection, and in xenograft rejection, RS-61443 may be superior to cyclosporine and FK 506 in these respects [13]. This effect may also prevent the generation of anti-OKT3 or (anti-thermocyte globulin) antibodies which lead to the failure of second use.

The studies have shown that the structural and compositional changes in the membranes of MPA-treated cells caused by disruption of the biosynthesis of cell surface receptors were associated with a marked reduction in antigen-binding sites and suppression of cell agglutination by concanavalin A [14].

The transfer of mannose and fucose to glycoprotein occurs through guanosine diphosphate intermediates bound to dolichol phosphate. Depletion of GTP would be expected to inhibit the transfer of mannose and fucose to glycoprotein, including adhesion molecules.

Treatment of either T cells or IL-1-activated endothelial cells with MPA in therapeutically attainable doses decreased lymphocyte attachment, and when both cell types were treated with MPA, the attachment was further inhibited [15].

During the past few years, the adhesion molecules which promote adhesion of various classes of white blood cells to vascular endothelium have been considered to play an important role in the immune response. Intercellular adhesion molecule-1 (ICAM-1) and vascular cell adhesion molecule-1 (VCAM-1) of endothelial cells are immunoglobulin superfamily adhesion receptors. ICAM-1 is the counterreceptor for lymphocyte function-associated antigen-1 (LFA-1) which is a member of the integrin family and expresses on T and B lymphocytes. Similarly,

VCAM-1 reacts with very late antigen-4 (VLA-4), a β-1 integrin expressed on resting lymphocytes and monocytes [16].

Endothelial cells exposed to cytokines may result in enhanced expression and receptor activity of adhesion molecules. Cytokine-stimulated endothelium becomes adhesive for leukocytes [17].

Interaction between the lymphocytes subset are involved in adhesion molecules. B lymphocytes express high levels of LFA-1 (CD11a/18) and VLA-4 (CD49d), white is oil antigen-presenting cells express high levels of adhesion receptors ICAM-1 (CD54) and VCAM-1 during the activation. This process is considered to be a control step in the generation of memory B cells [18].

The prevalence of ICAM-1 and VCAM-1 expression has been found in the cardiac allograft biopsy specimens. ICAM-1 was commonly present in heart biopsy with or without rejection. VCAM-1, on the other hand, was present much more commonly in the heart biopsy specimens with rejection [19]. Anti-ICAM-1 (R6.5) has been demonstrated to prolong graft survival in renal transplant in the animal models [20]. It has also showed a reversing effect on the ongoing rejection [21]. The same results have been achieved by monoclonal antibody against human T-cell adhesion molecules LFA-1. In vitro, monoclonal antibodies against ICAM-1 and VCAM-1 displayed inhibitory effects on the adherence between endothelial cells and lymphocytes [22].

It is also attractive to postulate a connection between the expression of adhesion molecules causing migration of lymphocytes across endothelium in rejection and the accumulation of subendothelial monocytes in presumably rejection-related atherosclerosis. Cybulsky and Gimbrone in Boston [23] have demonstrated evidence of a VCAM-like molecules in developing atherosclerotic plaques in rabbits model.

Because adhesion molecules may play a critical role in the allograft rejection, inhibition of the expression of such molecules could block the rejection process. The expression of adhesion molecules requires transfer of mannose and fucose to glycoprotein through guanosine diphosphate intermediates bound to dolichol phosphate; therefore, RS-61443 would be expected to inhibit the synthesis of adhesion molecules.

In vivo studies have demonstrated that RS-61443 can prolong the skin graft [27], pancreas graft [24], renal graft [26], and heart graft [25]. Combined with a small dose of cyclosporine A, RS-61443 could prolong the graft survival without side effects [26]. RS-61443 has also displayed reversing effect on the ongoing rejection [30]. The donor-specific immune tolerance has been induced by RS-61443 in animal models [28]. Although the immunosuppressive effect is stronger when combined with cyclosporine A, the tolerance-inducing effect was less effective when combined with cyclosporine A; the mechanism remains unknown. Prevention of the graft rejection in the presensitized recipient by RS-61443 has been demonstrated. Although the clinical trial did not lead the conclusion, the results were encouraging [29].

In summary, RS-61443 is a novel immunosuppressive drug acting on both T and B lymphocytes with a profile of activities distinct from those of cyclosporine and FK 506. Further understanding of the effects of RS-61443 on the B lymphocyte activation and the adhesion molecules will be necessary.

METHODS AND MATERIAL

In Vitro Assay

The effects of RS-61443 on the expression of VCAM-1 and ICAM-1 of endothelial cells. Endothelial cells will be obtained from human umbilical cord veins by the method of Maruyama and cultured in TC 199 containing 20% hcat-inactivated fetal bovine serum (FBS), penicillin (200 U/ml), streptomycin (200 µg/ml), and L-glutamine (2 mM) with and without RS-61443 [dissolved in dimethyl sulfoxide (10^{-2} mol/L) and diluted in culture medium in the concentration range 10^{-9} to 10^{-5} mol/L] at 37°C under 5% CO_2. Second to fourth passage confluent cultures of HUVEC will be used, as there was no difference in ICAM-1 expression by inactivated versus activated high umbilical vein endothelial cells (HUVEC) between primary and fourth passage cultures. HUVEC will be incubated for 6 h at 37°C in 5% CO_2 with 5 U/ml cell-derived IL-1 (GUPI 1A, Genzyme, Boston, MA), 100 ng/ml LPS (E. coli, 055:B5, Sigma), 100 U/ml rhTNF-alpha (Genzyme), or PBS. ICAM-1 and VCAM-1 expression by HUVEC will be quantitated by using anti-ICAM-1 (RR1) and anti-VCAM-1 monoclonal antibodies which will be determined by enzyme-linked immunosorbent assay (ELISA). Anti-MHC-I and anti-MHC-II monoclonal antibodies will be used to detect MHC-I and MHC-II antigens expression, respectively. The adherence assay will be performed following the details described later.

The effects of RS-61443 on the expression of LFA-1 and VLA-4 on the B and T lymphocytes. The spleen from the organ donor (ethic approval will be obtained) will be passed through 701 nylon mesh, layered and centrifuged on ficoll-hypaque (Sigma), and cultured in RPMI 1640 medium supplemented with 20% human serum, 10 mM HEPES solution, and 100 U/ml penicillin, 100 mg/ml streptomycin. B lymphocytes will be separated using the rosett technique. The splenocyte will be incubated with or without RS-61443 (concentration described as above) and stimulators for 3 days. One group of splenocytes will be treated by RS-61443 for 24 before incubating with a stimulator. The stimulator will be an irradiated splenocyte (MLC), PHA, and pokeweed mitogen (PWM) 20 ug/ml or IL-4. Cyclosporine A and FK 506 will be used as controls. LFA-1 and VLA-4 expression will be quantitated by using anti-LAF-1 (CD11a/CD18) and anti-VLA-4 (CD49d/CD29) monoclonal antibodies which will be determined by flow cytometry assay (technique details described separately). CD3, CD4, CD8, CD23, anti-MHC II, and anti-IgM monoclonal antibodies will be used to detect surface antigens. The effects of RS-61443 on the proliferation response of T and B lymphocytes to various stimulators will be tested by the uptake of tritiated thymidine (details see the subsection In Vivo assay, Axial Lymphocyte Culture).

Flow cytometry assay. The target cells will be prepared and washed in the Hank's medium with 2% heat-inactivated fetal bovine serum (FBS), adjusted to 2×10^7/ml in Hank's medium with 10% FBS and incubated at 37°C for 20 min to minimize nonspecific antibody binding. The cells (5×10^5 in 25μl) will be incubated with 20 μl monoclonal antibodies (various dilution) at room temperature for 20 min, washed twice to remove unbounded antibody, then incubated with second antibodies conjugated with FITC or PE. The cells will be washed once and fixed in FACS fixative and analyzed using a flow cytometer.

Adherence assay. RS-61443-treated and -untreated HUVEC cells (stimulated by IL-1 or rhTNF-alpha) will be plated onto gelatin-coated 48-well tissue culture plates and allowed to reach confluence. The medium will be decanted and the well will be washed twice with RPMI containing 2% NCS. Subsequently, RS-61443-treated and -untreated splenocyte (^{51}Cr labeled) will be added to each well. Following 30 min incubation at 37°C, nonadherent cells will be discarded and the wells will be washed once with 0.5 ml PBS. Adherent cells will be lysed with 1 N NH4OH and the lysate will be collected and counted in a gamma spectrophotometer. Percent adherence will be calculated by the formula

$$\frac{\text{cpm in lysate}}{\text{cpm total release}}$$

In Vivo assay

Animal model. Mature, inbred LBN (RT-1) will be used as recipient and syngeneic donor. ACI (RT-1) will serve as an allogeneic donor.

Every group includes six animals. Experimental groups will be dosed orally with RS-61443 80 mg/kg only once a day from day -1 to day 30 relative to the time of graft, with RS-61443 and cyclosporine A, and with cyclosporine A only. All the experiments will be carried out with the approval of the Institute Animal Care and Use Committee. The research will strictly follow the current *Guide for the Care and Use of Laboratory Animals* (NIH publication, DHHS/USPHS) and federal laws and regulations.

Operation technique.   The donor animal will be anaesthetized using Rompum (Glaxo) 3mg/kg and Ketamine (Park-Davis) 60mg/kg intramuscularly. The veins will be ligated. The heart with ascending aorta and pulmonary artery will be dissected out under clean condition. The recipient animal will be anaesthetized using the same technique as described. Laparotomy will be performed. The heart will be grafted heterotopiclly into the infrarenal abdominal aorta and inferior vena cava of the recipient. The end-to-side anastomosis will be performed using continuous 10-0 nylon sutures for donor aorta to recipient aorta and donor pulmonary artery to recipient IVC. The laparotomy will be closed using continuous proline suture. The grafted heart will be checked by abdominal palpation daily. Disappearance of contraction will be regarded as total rejection. All the experimental animals will be closely observed postoperatively by the investigators. The rats will be put in the warm cage. The breath and heart rate will be checked every 2 until anaesthetic recovery. The animals will be sacrificed under the anaesthesia. The spleen, heart, and serum will be collected for immunology and histology studies.

Preparation of spleen cells.   The spleen will be passed through 701 nylon mesh, layered, and centrifuged (2000 rpm) on lymphocyte rat ficoll-paque (C5054, Cedarland Laboratories Limited). The lymphocyte will be collected and washed twice with completed medium (RPMI 1640 supplemented with 2 mM L-glutamine, 10 mM HEPES solution, 5×10^{-5} M 2-mercaptoethanol (2-ME), 100 U/ml penicillin, 100 mg/ml streptomycin, and 10% heat-inactivated fetal bovine serum).

Mixed lymphocyte culture.   Stimulator and responder splenocytes will be prepared as described above. The responder will be collected from the recipient. The stimulator will come from the donor strain and irradiated with 2500 rads. Whistart strain will serve as third-party cells. One-way mixed lymphocyte culture will be carried out in 96-well, round-bottomed microtiter plates. Replicated culture including 1×10^5 responder and 1×10^5 stimulator will be incubated for 5 days at 37°C in

95% air, 5% CO_2. Each well will be pulsed with 1 μCi tritiated thymidine for 18 h prior to harvesting. Radioactivity will be measured in a scintillation counter. The stimulation index will be calculated by the formula

$$SI = \frac{cpm\ autologous}{cpm\ experimental}$$

Cytotoxic assay. The cytotoxicity of lymphocytes will be quantitated in spleen cells isolated from heart allograft recipients. Target cells will be prepared by culturing donor-strain spleen cells under standard condition for 2 days with Con-A (2 mg/ml). The Con-A blasts will be collected, adjusted to 1×10^7 cells/100 μl, incubated with 100 μCi ^{51}Cr for 60 min and gently washed three times before use. MLC will be prepared as described above. After 8 days of incubation, the cytotoxic activity of each well will be assessed by an additional 6 h incubation at 37°C with ^{51}Cr-labeled target cells (effector:target = 20:1 to 5:1). The supernants (100 μl) will be harvested and measured in a gamma counter. The cytotoxicity will be calculated by the formula:

$$\frac{(cpm\ experimental\ -\ cpm\ spontaneous)}{(cpm\ total\ release\ -\ cmp\ spontaneous)}$$

Antidonor specific antibodies (flow cytometry assay). Splenocytes of the donor strain will be used as target cells and Whistart strain as third-party control to examine for donor-specific alloantibodies generation following heart allograft. The cells will be incubated with recipient serum and second antibody (goat antirat IgG-FITC, ICN 67-242). For the technique details see the Subsection In Vitro Assay, Flow Cytometry Assay.

Expression of adhesion molecules on the T and B lymphocytes from heart allograft recipient. Splenocyte of recipient will be prepared as described above. The cells will incubated with CD11a/18 (LFA-1), CD49d/CD29 (VLA-4), CD19, CD23, anti-IgM, CD3, CD4 and CD8 monoclonal antibodies. The samples will be tested on flow cytometer (details in the Subsection In Vitro Assay, Flow Cytometry Assay).

Prevention of sensitization of OKT3 and ATG by RS-61443. The animals will be injected with OKT3 or ATG for 7–14 days. Experimental groups will be dosed with RS-61443 only, RS-61443 with cyclosporine A, and cyclosporine A only. OKT3 and ATG injection only will serve as control. The serum are collected for flow cytometry assay. The mouse lymphocytes are used as targets reacted with serum from experiment animal and secondary antirat antibody conjugated with FITC. The samples are tested in a flow cytometer (details see in the Subsection In Vitro Assay, Flow Cytometry Assay).

Histology and immunohistology studies.   The transplanted heart will be collected and snap-frozen in OCT compound. The sections will be stained by hematoxylin–eosin and elastic–Van Gieson stain. Anti-ICAM-1, anti-VCAM-1, CD11a/18, CD49d/29, CD4, and CD8 monoclonal antibodies will be used for immunohistology studies.

Statistical analysis.   Comparisons between the group will be made using the Student's *t*-test.

ETHICAL CONSIDERATION OF THE RESEARCH

This study will involve the human materials and rat. Approval from Institute Ethic Committee and Animal Care and Use Committee will be obtained and carefully watched. All the experimental animals will receive individualized human care for the duration of the study. The postoperative period will be observed carefully by the investigators until anaesthetic recovery.

REFERENCES

1. Kriett JM, Kaye MP. The registry of the international society for heart transplantation: Seventh official report—1990. *J Heart Lung Transplant* 1990;9:323–330.
2. Uretsky BF, Murali S, Reddy PS. Development of coronary artery disease in cardiac transplantation patients receiving immunosuppressive therapy with cyclosporine and prednisone. *Circulation* 1987;76:827–833.
3. Billingham ME. Cardiac transplant atherosclerosis. *Transplant Proc* 1987;19(Suppl. 5):19–25.
4. Hammond EH, Ensley RD, Yowell RL. Vascular rejection of human cardiac allograft and the role of human immunity in chronic allograft rejection. *Transplant Proc* 1991;23(Suppl. 2):26–30.
5. Hosenpud JD, Shipley GD, Wagner CR. Cardiac allograft vasculopathy: Current concepts, recent developments and future directions. *J Heart Lung Transplant* 1992;11:9–23.
6. Nelson PH, Eugui E, Wang CC. Synthesis and immunosuppressive activity of some side-chain variants of mycophenolic acid. *J Med Chem* 1990;33:833.

7. Allison AC, Hovi T. *Ciba Found Symp* 1977;48:207.

8. Nguyen BT, Sadee W. Compartmentation of guanine nucleotide precursors for DNA synthesis. *Biochem J* 1986;234:263.

9. Lucas DL, Webster HK. *J Clin Invest* 1983;72:1889.

10. Rigley K, Harnett M. In: Callard RC, ed. *Cytokines and B Lymphocytes.* Academic Press, San Diego: 1990, 41.

11. Grailer A, Nichols J, Hullett D. Inhibition of human B cell responses in vitro by RS-61443, cyclosporine A and DAB486-IL-2. *Transplant Proc* 1991;23:314–315.

12. Burlingham WJ, Grailer AP, Hullett DA. Inhibition of both MLC and in vitro IgG memory response to tetanus toxoid by RS-61443. *Transplantation* 1991;51:545–547.

13. Knechtle SJ, Wang J, Burlingham WJ. The influence of RS-61443 on antibody-mediated rejection. *Transplantation* 1992;53:699–701.

14. Sokoloski JA, Sartorelli AC. *Mol Pharmacol* 1985;28:567.

15. Allison AC, Almquist SJ, Muller CD. In vitro immunosuppressive effects of mycophenolic acid and an ester pro-drug, RS-61443. *Transplant Proc* 1991;23(Suppl. 2):10.

16. Springer TA. Adhesion receptors of the immune system. *Nature* 1990;346:425–434.

17. Suciu-foca N, Reed E, Marboe C. The role of anti-HLA antibodies in heart transplantation. *Transplantation* 1991;51:716–724.

18. Koopman G, Parmentier HK, Schuurman HJ. Adhesion of human B cells to follicular dendritic cells involves both the lymphocyte function-associated antigen 1/intercellular adhesion molecule 1 and very late antigen 4/vascular cell adhesion molecule 1 pathways. *J Exp Med* 1991;173:1297–1304.

19. Allen MD, McDonald TO, Carlos T. Endothelial adhesion molecules in heart transplantation. *J Heart Lung Transplant* 1992;11:S8–S13.

20. Cosimi AB, Conti D, Delmonico FL. In vivo effects of monoclonal antibody to ICAM-1 (CD54) in nonhuman primates with renal allografts. *J Immunol* 1990;144:4604–4612.

21. Wee LS, Cosimi AB, Preffer FI. Functional consequences of anti-ICAM-1 (CD54) in cynomolgus monkeys with renal allografts. *Transplant Proc* 1991;23:279–280.

22. Berlin PJ, Bacher JD, Sharrow SO. Monoclonal antibodies against human T cell adhesion molecules—modulation of immune function in nonhuman primates. *Transplantation* 1992;53:840–849.

23. Cybulsky MI, Gimbrone MA. Endothelial expression of a mononuclear leukocyte adhesion molecule during atherogenesis. *Science* 1991;251:788–791.

24. Coulombe M, Hao L, Calcinaro F. Tolerance induction in adult animals: Comparison of RS-61443 and anti-CD4 treatment. *Transplant Proc* 1991;23(Suppl. 2):31–32.

25. Morris RE, Hoyt EG, Murphy MP. Mycophenolic acid morpholinoe-

thylester (RS-61443) is a new immunosuppressant that prevents and halts heart allograft rejection by selective inhibition of T and B cell purine synthesis. *Transplant Proc* 1990;22:1659–1662.

26. Platz KP, Sollinger HW, Hullett DA. RS-61443 a new, potent immunosuppressive agent. *Transplantation* 1991;51:27–30.

27. Platz KP, Eckhoff DE, Hullett DA. Prolongation of dog renal allograft survival by RS-61443, a new, potent immunosuppressive agent. *Transplant Proc* 1991;23:497–498.

28. Morris RE, Wang J. Effect of splenectomy and mono- or combination therapy with rapamycin, the morpholonoethyl ester of mycophenolic acid and deoxyspergualin on cardiac xenograft survival. *Transplant Proc* 1991;23:699–702.

29. Sollinger HW, Deierhoi MH, Belzer FO. RS-61443 a phase I clinical trial and pilot rescue study. *Transplantation* 1992;53:428–432.

30. Platz KP, Bechstein WO, Eckhoff DE. RS-61443 reverses acute allograft rejection in dogs. *Surgery* 1991;110(4):736–741.

13

Cardiac Transplantation in the Elderly: Emerging Ethical Issues

Mark D. Fox

This case discussion will differ from others in this volume in that it will focus primarily on the ethical issues posed by a case presentation from the clinical practice of transplantation.

CASE PRESENTATION

A 67-year-old white male with a history of idiopathic dilated cardiomyopathy (IDC), chronic atrial fibrillation (AF), and congestive heart failure (CHF) presented to the Heart Failure and Transplantation Program in the fall of 1992 for transplant evaluation. The patient had been followed by a local cardiologist since presenting with atrial fibrillation in 1986. He underwent DC cardioversion and was maintained in normal sinus rhythm on quinidine until he became intolerant of it. In August 1990, the patient was again in AF when admitted to a local hospital with congestive heart failure.

The patient was rehospitalized in December 1990 with CHF requiring increased diuresis. Cardiac catheterization at that time revealed normal coronary arteries, pulmonary artery (PA) pressure of 50/20 mm Hg, pulmonary capillary wedge pressure (PCWP) 18 mm Hg, and cardiac output 4.4 L/min, with an ejection fraction (EF) of 0.25–0.30. The patient was referred for transplant evaluation in January 1991 at the age of 65 years. Echocardiography revealed a dilated left ventricle, bilateral atrial enlargement, mild mitral regurgitation, and trivial tricuspid regurgitation. In view of his chronic AF, the patient was loaded with procainamide and underwent repeat DC cardioversion; however, this attempt failed to maintain normal sinus rhythm.

The patient was declined as a candidate for cardiac transplantation because of his relatively stable condition and advanced age. When his symptoms worsened, the patient sought evaluation for cardiomyoplasty at another center. The patient declined the procedure and returned home on medical management for IDC and CHF.

The patient was referred once again for transplant evaluation in the fall of 1992. He underwent a thorough transplant evaluation with echocardiography, cardiac catheterization, pulmonary function testing, blood chemistries and serologies, and a psychosocial evaluation by the transplant social worker. Repeat catheterization revealed normal coronary arteries, moderately severe but reversible pulmonary hypertension with a PA pressure of 67/30 mm Hg, and an EF of 0.16. Despite his advanced age, the patient was felt to be a good candidate for cardiac transplantation in light of his otherwise excellent health, strong psychosocial support, and personal motivation. He was placed on the United Network for Organ Sharing (UNOS) waiting list in October 1992.

The patient was admitted in November 1992 with increasing dyspnea, dyspnea on exertion, and three-pillow orthopnea. He was treated with dopamine and dobutamine and remained hospitalized on pressors until February 1993, when he underwent orthotopic cardiac transplantation.

DISCUSSION

Age limits for cardiac transplantation have been extended at both ends of the life spectrum over the last several years. Heart transplantation is now successfully performed in infants and neonates; in fact, it is now acceptable to place fetuses on the waiting list for cardiac transplantation.

The upper age limit of eligibility for transplantation has been extended as well. In 1982, the cardiac transplant program at Stanford reported age 50 as the upper limit of their recipient selection criteria [1]. However, by 1986 the criteria for Medicare coverage for heart transplantation cited the "mid-50s" (age 53–57) as the recommended age limit for recipient selection [2]. The continued evolution of the upper age limit for cardiac transplantation is well demonstrated in the case of the patient presented. He was declined for transplantation at age 65 due in part to advanced age but was subsequently accepted (at the same institution) and transplanted 2 years later.

Transplant Candidacy and the Elderly

Data from the United Network for Organ Sharing (UNOS) and the International Society for Heart and Lung Transplantation (ISHLT) reflect the extension of the upper age limit for transplantation in recent years. According to ISHLT registry data, the number of cardiac transplants in elderly patients has increased 10-fold over the last 6 years, from 9 in 1986 to 92 in 1992 (personal communication, ISHLT Registry, 1993) (Fig. 13-1). In addition, the number of patients age 65 and older on the UNOS waiting list has continued to grow in each of the last 5 years (Fig. 13-2). In fact, the total number of patients awaiting cardiac transplantation has increased more than 150% since 1988, with a total of 2693 patients on the waiting list as of December 31, 1992 (personal communication, UNOS, 1993) (Fig. 13-3). However, during this same period, the number of transplants performed each year increased by only 30%, from 1675 transplants in 1988 to 2173 in 1992 (personal communication, UNOS, 1993) (Fig. 13-3).

Transplantation in Patients Age 65 and over

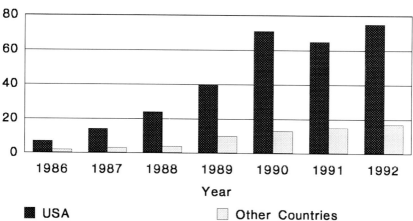

Figure 13-1. Number of cardiac transplantation procedures performed in patients age 65 and older, in the United States and other countries, 1986–1993. (*Source*: ISHLT Registry.)

Patients Age 65 and over on UNOS Waiting List

Number of patients

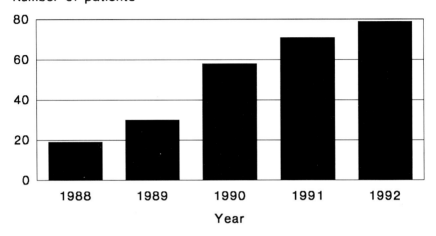

Figure 13-2.   Number of patients age 65 and older on UNOS waiting list for cardiac transplantation at year end, 1988–1992. (*Source*: UNOS.)

Growth in Waiting List vs. Transplants Performed

Number of patients

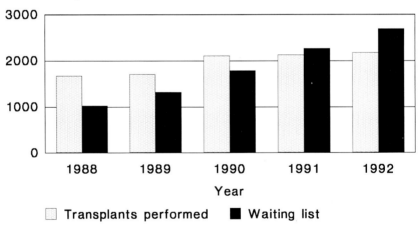

Figure 13-3.   Total number of cardiac transplants performed and total number of patients awaiting cardiac transplantation at year end in the United States, 1988–1992. (*Source*: UNOS.)

Although the absolute number of patients age 65 and over on the waiting list has increased in recent years, the elderly have constituted a relatively constant proportion of the total waiting list—approximately 2–3% (Fig. 13-4). Likewise, the elderly have remained a stable percentage of the total number of transplants performed, as well as the percentage of patients dying while on the waiting list (Fig. 13-4). These data suggest that elderly patients are being transplanted or dying while waiting in approximately equal proportion to the rate at which they are being listed for transplantation.

Although transplantation of the elderly has emerged as an acceptable practice in recent years, there has been considerable concern in the transplant community regarding the justification for considering the elderly for transplantation. Extending the age limit for transplantation has increased the pool of potential recipients while the donor pool has essentially plateaued. At present, more than 25% of patients awaiting cardiac transplantation die before a donor heart becomes available [3]. Thus, any expansion of the pool of potential recipients must be justified in light of the already-limited supply of organs. Other concerns regarding transplantation in the elderly have focused primarily on three issues: perioperative survival, longevity, and quality-life years. First, based on Stanford's early experience with 21 patients over

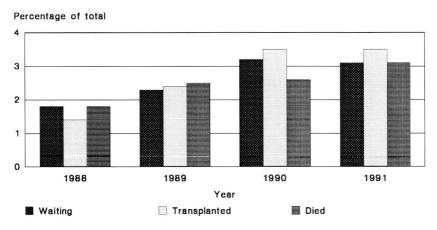

Figure 13-4. Patients age 65 and older as a percentage of all patients in each of three outcome categories: patients awaiting cardiac transplantation, patients transplanted, and patients dying while awaiting transplantation, for each year 1988–1991. (*Source*: UNOS.)

age 50, it was felt that older patients did not have the capacity to withstand postoperative complications [1]. Second, elderly patients may die of other causes before the graft ceases to function. In other words, the graft may outlive the patient. Finally, some argue that younger patients have more years to be productive and make use of the quality of life afforded by transplantation. To address these concerns, it is necessary to review the data on heart failure and transplantation in the elderly.

Heart Failure in the Elderly: A Brief Overview

The elderly represent the fastest-growing segment of the U.S. population. Twelve percent of the U.S. population was considered elderly (age 65 or older) in 1989 [4]; it is projected that this figure will approximately double by the year 2030 [5]. Congestive heart failure is the most common hospital discharge diagnosis in this population [6]. In addition, data from the Framingham Heart Study reveal that the annual incidence of CHF rises with advancing age [7, 8].

Prognosis for 142 patients with CHF in the original Framingham study was poor: 5-year survival following the onset of CHF was 38.5% for men and 56.7% for women [7]. A follow-up study [8] of 9405 subjects from the original Framingham cohort and the Framingham Offspring Study analyzed survival following the onset of CHF in 652 patients. Ho et al. [8] report 1- and 5-year survival rates of 57% and 25%, respectively for men, and 64% and 38%, respectively, for women. However, for those patients surviving at least 90 days after the onset of CHF (a sample comparable to that selected for most heart failure intervention trials), 1-year survival improved to 79% for men and 88% for women. Five-year survival also improved for this population, to 35% in men and 53% in women [8].

Other researchers have correlated survival with New York Heart Association (NYHA) functional class. Survival rates for patients in NYHA Class I to III were 75% at 1 year and 48% at 5 years [9]. Prognosis was even more dismal for patients in NYHA Class IV, with a 1-year mortality rate of approximately 50% [9]. Results from the Cooperative North Scandinavian Enalapril Survival Study (CONSENSUS) [10] were similar for patients in NYHA Class IV. Probability of survival at 1 year for 126 patients treated with conventional heart failure therapy and placebo was 37%. Treatment with enalapril and conventional therapy improved the probability of survival at 1 year to approximately 55% in a sample of 127 patients [10].

It is clear from these data that a large number of elderly patients could benefit from transplantation. However, the prevalence of co-morbid chronic disease at initial diagnosis of CHF is roughly 60% [7]. Thus, not all older patients with advanced CHF would be suitable candidates for transplantation. Furthermore, survival data are not segregated for patients with or without other chronic illnesses. In addition, the prevalence of other chronic disease for specific age-group cohorts is not reported in the Framingham data. It is not possible, then, to anticipate the actual numbers of elderly patients with CHF but no other chronic disease who might, thus, be suitable transplant candidates; nor is it possible to predict survival for elderly patients with CHF who are otherwise free of chronic disease. Inasmuch as the elderly are the fastest growing segment of the population, it is reasonable to anticipate that the numbers of elderly patients who would be potential transplant candidates will continue to grow.

Transplantation in the Elderly

Several centers have reported series of patients transplanted beyond their previously established age criteria (Table 13-1) [11–20]. Seven of the earliest studies report actuarial survival following transplantation in elderly patients equal to or better than that found in the younger group of patients [11–16, 18]. However, several more recent studies contradict these data, two for cohorts of patients age 55 or older, the other for patients age 65 or older [17, 19, 20]. Only one study demonstrated

Table 13-1. Summary of 10 Published Reports on Cardiac Transplantation in Patients Older than a Previously Established Age Limit

First Author	Year	Age	N	One-Year Actuarial Survival Older vs. Younger Cohort
Carrier	1986	50	13	72% vs. 66%
Renlund	1987	54	21	100% vs. 94%
Frazier	1988	60	28	83% vs. 75%
Miller	1988	55	8	100% vs. 82%[a]
Olivari	1988	55	23	96% vs. 96%
Aravot	1989	60	25	84%[b]
Hosenpud	1990	55	20	77% vs. 87%
Amrein	1990	55	31	91% vs. 84%
Fabbri	1992	55	46	72% vs. 87%[c]
Heroux	1993	65	12	71% vs. 87%

[a]Gross survival through average follow-up of 10.4 months.

[b]Actuarial survival for patients over age 60; no younger cohort.

[c]These percentages are estimates extrapolated from a graph of actuarial survival; differences in survival were significant at $p < .05$.

a statistically significant difference in survival; Fabbri et al. represent graphically a decreased actuarial survival in patients age 55 and older that is significant at the $p < .05$ level [19]. Cumulative data from the ISHLT registry reveal survival rates following transplantation in elderly patients equal to or better than all other age groups (personal communication, UNOS, 1993) (Fig. 13-5); likewise, the UNOS data reflect survival rates in patients age 65 and older comparable to those achieved in younger patients [3]. It is unclear, however, to what extent these data can be extrapolated to patients beyond the age of 65.

Furthermore, it is important to recognize that survival data for elderly patients represent a smaller sample size than is available for other age groups. Nevertheless, several factors may be beneficial for elderly patients as compared to other age cohorts with regard to survival posttransplant. First, elderly patients are likely more carefully screened than younger patients, and those with significant risk factors may be declined for transplantation. In the case presented, the patient had essentially no co-morbidity. Further, data suggest that elderly patients experience fewer rejection episodes than their younger counterparts. Several series report a statistically significant decreased incidence of allograft rejection in older patients [12, 20]. Similarly, acute rejection accounts for a lower proportion of posttransplant hospital admissions in elderly patients than in their younger counterparts [17]. Thus, immu-

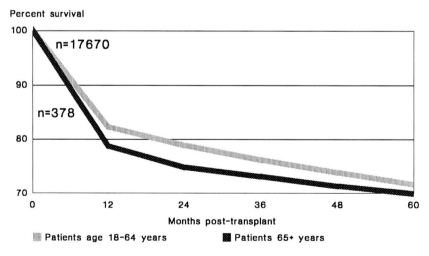

Actuarial Survival Post-Transplant

Figure 13-5. Actuarial survival following cardiac transplantation for patients age 18–64 years and for patients age 65 years and older. (*Source*: ISHLT Registry.)

nosenescence may make elderly patients less prone to the morbidity and mortality associated with severe rejection and its treatment.

Despite their decreased morbidity due to graft rejection, elderly patients may be at higher risk for morbidity due to other causes. There appears to be a higher incidence of infectious complications in elderly transplant recipients; two institutions report a statistically significant increase in infectious episodes in their elderly cohort of patients [15, 20]. In addition, Amrein et al. report a significantly increased incidence ($p < .001$) of gastrointestinal complications in their series of 31 patients age 55 and older [18]. Further, these gastrointestinal complications were associated with higher mortality in elderly patients in the first month posttransplant. Beyond the immediate perioperative period, however, the older patients had a significantly decreased ($p \le .05$) mortality rate when compared with their younger counterparts [18].

Life Expectancy and Long-Term Survival

Concerns about longevity in elderly transplant recipients relate to overall life expectancy. As of 1989, the average life expectancy at birth in the United States was 71.8 years for men and 78.6 years for women [4]. Thus, patients transplanted at age 65 initially appear to have an additional life expectancy of only 6.8 years and 13.6 years for men and women, respectively. However, the additional life expectancies for those individuals who survive to age 65 are 15.2 years for men and 18.8 years for women [4]. These data must be weighed against the backdrop of the expected graft survival for hearts transplanted today, which has not yet been well defined. Long-term survival data from the ISHLT registry reveal 10-year actuarial survival of 59.5% for all adult patients transplanted (excluding retransplants) from 1967 to 1992 (personal communication, ISHLT registry, 1993). Transplantation in patients age 65 and over is a more recent phenomenon; nevertheless, 7-year survival following heart transplantation in elderly patients has been calculated at 58.7% (personal communication, ISHLT registry, 1993). Thus, based on the long-term graft survival data and the additional life expectancy for individuals at age 65, the claim that grafts in elderly patients may outlive the recipient cannot be supported.

Societal Values and the Need for Consensus

These data demonstrate that transplantation in elderly patients may result in survival rates following transplantation comparable to those achieved in younger patients. The third concern expressed in regard to transplantation in the elderly surrounds the quality-life years remaining to elderly patients. Although data on life expectancy suggest that elderly patients may have 15 years or longer of anticipated survival, the crux of this issue revolves around what constitutes "quality?"; that is, what defines a successful outcome in transplantation? One may attempt to address this issue via rehabilitation data regarding functional capacity, exercise tolerance, or return to work. Others might rely on patient reports of quality of life. Patient and graft survival clearly must be considerations in defining successful outcomes following transplantation; similarly, functional capacity has a place in this assessment. Beyond these criteria, however, there is no consensus regarding the goals and expectations of transplantation. To address adequately the issues surrounding transplantation in the elderly will require the much broader effort of developing a societal understanding of the appropriate goals in undertaking transplantation. Similarly, the current effort to reform health care requires a broader consensus regarding the status of transplantation, in terms of both the expectations of health and health care and the appropriations decisions regarding health care expenditures.

In a similar way, the related issues of societal expectations and consensus surround the practice of transplantation in the elderly, and health care for the elderly more generally. A variety of ethical issues and policy concerns arise from this prevailing ambiguity. Concerns regarding what constitutes appropriate care for the aged arise from an ambivalence about the status of the elderly in our society. Furthermore, concerns about what expectations for health are reasonable, particularly in the elderly, reflect an anxiety surrounding the natural processes of aging, decline, and death. Thus, the challenge of health care reform generally and the care of the elderly specifically rests on the resolution of the fundamental ambivalence of societal values regarding health, aging, and death.

ACKNOWLEDGMENTS

The authors acknowledge with gratitude the assistance of Gottlieb C. Friesinger, M.D. in clarifying the issues presented in this chapter.

REFERENCES

1. Pennock JL, Oyer PE, Reitz BA et al. Cardiac transplantation in perspective for the future: Survival, complications, rehabilitation, and cost. *J Thorac Cardiovasc Surg* 1982;83:168–177.

2. Medicare Program; criteria for Medicare coverage of heart transplants. *Federal Reg.* 1986;51:37164–37170.

3. *1993 Annual Report of the U.S. Scientific Registry for Transplant Recipients and the Organ Procurement and Transplantation Network—Transplant Data: 1988–1991.* UNOS; Richmond, VA; and Division of Organ Transplantation, Bureau of Health Resources Development, Health Resources and Services Administration, U.S. Department of Health and Human Services, 1993.

4. National Center for Health Statistics. *Health, United States, 1991.* Hyattsville, MD: Public Health Service, 1992.

5. Tighe D, Brest AN. Congestive heart failure in the elderly. In: Lowenthal DT, ed. *Geriatric Cardiology.* Philadelphia: F.A. Davis, 1992:127–138.

6. Parmley WW. Pathophysiology and current therapy of congestive heart failure. *J Am Coll Cardiol* 1989;13:771–785.

7. McKee PA, Castelli WP, McNamara PM, Kannel WB. The natural history of congestive heart failure: The Framingham study. *N Engl J Med* 1971;285:1441–1446.

8. Ho KKL, Pinsky JL, Kannel WB, Levy D. The epidemiology of heart failure: The Framingham study. *J Am Coll Cardiol* 1993;22(Suppl. A):6A–13A.

9. Smith WM. Epidemiology of congestive heart failure. *Am J Cardiol* 1985;55:3A–8A.

10. The CONSENSUS Trial Study Group. Effects of enalapril on mortality in severe congestive heart failure: Results of the Cooperative North Scandinavian Enalapril Survival Study (CONSENSUS). *N Engl J Med* 1987;316:1429–1435.

11. Carrier M, Emery RW, Riley JE, Levinson MM, Copeland JG. Cardiac transplantation in patients over 50 years of age. *J Am Coll Cardiol* 1986;8:285–288.

12. Renlund DG, Gilbert EM, O'Connell JB et al. Age-associated decline in cardiac allograft rejection. *Am J Med* 1987;83:391–398.

13. Frazier OH, Macris MP, Duncan JM, Van Buren CT, Cooley DA. Cardiac transplantation in patients over 60 years of age. *Ann Thorac Surg* 1988;45:129–132.

14. Miller LW, Vitale-Noedel N, Pennington DG, McBride L, Kanter KR. Heart transplantation in patients over age 55 years. *J Heart Transplant* 1988;7:254–257.

15. Olivari MT, Antolick A, Kaye MP, Jamieson SW, Ring WS. Heart transplantation in elderly patients. *J Heart Transplant* 1988;7:258–264.

16. Aravot DJ, Banner NR, Khaghani A et al. Cardiac transplantation in the seventh decade of life. *Am J Cardiol* 1989;63:90–93.

17. Hosenpud JD, Pantely GA, Norman DJ, Cobanoglu AM, Hovaguimian H, Starr A. A critical analysis of morbidity and mortality as it relates to recipient age following cardiac transplantation. *Clin Transplant* 1990;4:51–54.

18. Amrein C, Vulser C, Farge D et al. Is heart transplantation a valid therapy in elderly patients? *Transplant Proc* 1990;22:1454–1456.
19. Fabbri A, Sharples LD, Mullins P, Caine N, Large S, Wallwork J. Heart transplantation in patients over 54 years of age with triple-drug therapy immunosuppression. *J Heart Lung Transplant* 1992;11:929–932.
20. Heroux AL, Costanzo-Nordin MR, O'Sullivan JE et al. Heart transplantation as a treatment option for end-stage heart disease in patients older than 65 years of age. *J Heart Lung Transplant* 1993;12:573–579.

14

A Patient with New Onset Dyspnea and Airflow Obstruction at 4 Months after Combined Heart–Lung Transplantation for Eisenmenger's Syndrome

James E. Loyd and William H. Frist

CASE PRESENTATION

History of Present Illness

A 35-year-old white female was admitted 4 months after heart–lung transplantation for illness during the last 2 days; her symptoms included nausea, vomiting, malaise, and low-grade fever. She was Class IV NYHA before transplantation, and her transplant hospitalization was prolonged, but she had done well at home for the prior 2 months, walking a mile daily. She had a chronic nonproductive cough which was unchanged, but she now also described dyspnea with exertion.

Medications

The medications were as follows:

Cyclosporin 100 mg bid
Imuran 50 mg daily
Prednisone 15 mg daily

Zantac 150 mg bid
Lasix 80 mg daily
Septra DS one bid on Mondays

Examination

Examination of the patient presented the following:

T = 100.2°F; BP = 148/88; P = 106; RR = 22
35-year-old white female with cushingoid face
Head, ears, eyes, nose, throat: normal.
Lungs: rales at both lung bases
Cardiac: regular rhythm, without murmur or gallop
Abdomen: liver 1 cm below costal margin, nontender
Extremities: no edema

Laboratory

The laboratory results were as follows:

Hb   14.0 g%
Hct   40.1%
WBC 9.4×10^3 cells/mm^3
           85% PMN, 8% lymphs, 4% monos, 1% EOS
Platelets 328,000
Chemistries normal except BUN = 27, Cr = 1.6
ABG = pH = 7.47 pCO$_2$ = 41, pO$_2$ = 61

Chest radiography revealed median sternotomy wires, slightly elevated left hemidiaphragm, normal cardiac size, mild increase in interstitial pulmonary markings

Fiberoptic bronchoscopy was performed under local anesthesia and revealed a well-healed tracheal anastomosis. Bronchoalveolar lavage of the right lobe yielded 65% macrophages, 30% lymphocytes, and 5% neutrophils. Special stains and cytomegalovirus cultures were negative. Histology revealed mild focal acute inflammation.

Endomyocardial biopsy revealed mild acute rejection.

PRIOR MEDICAL HISTORY

Her medical history included dyspnea first noted during her only pregnancy at age 18, but a murmur had been noted since birth. Cardiac cath at age 18 showed pulmonary artery pressure of 94/43, mean 63 mm Hg with right-to-left intracardiac shunt, and pulmonary vascular resistance of 5.5 Woods units. A secundum atrial septal defect was repaired at age 24 and she noted transient clinical improvement in her dyspnea. Dyspnea and exertional limitations began progressive worsening at age 30, and increasing cardiomegaly was detected on chest radiograph. Cardiac catheterization revealed a pulmonary artery pressure of 73/33, mean = 47 mm Hg, and pulmonary vascular resistance of 5.5 Wood units. By age 33 she was chairbound and barely able to perform self-care. She had marked fatique, and moderate discomfort in the right upper quadrant, with continuous nausea. Dyspnea, orthopnea, and angina were also present. Cardiac catheterization revealed pulmonary artery pressure of 117/55, mean = 73 mm Hg and Pulmonary vascular resistance of 12 wood units. Her condition continued to decline with worsening right heart failure and numerous hospitalizations at ages 33 and 34.

At age 35 in February 1988, en bloc heart–lung transplantation was performed after awaiting a donor for 8 months. The early postoperative course was complicated by excessive hemorrhage from thoracostomy tubes, requiring mediastinal exploration on the first postoperative day. Her recovery was delayed by episodes of moderately severe cardiac rejection at both 1 week and 1 month posttransplant, but she responded well to bolus solumedrol and was discharged from the hospital on day 64 on triple immunosuppression with cyclosporin, imuran, and prednisone.

HOSPITAL COURSE AND SUBSEQUENT FOLLOW-UP

Treatment with solumedrol 1 g I.V. daily for 3 days was associated with transient subjective improvement, and the patient was released from the hospital in a week. However, she never returned to her former level of function. At 5 months posttransplant FVC was 2.06 L (59%), FEV1 was 0.86 L (31%) FEV1/FVC = 41%, and TLC was 3.32 (68%). The dramatic reduction in airflow demonstrated in the fall of FEV1 from 1.99 L to 0.86 L never improved during her later course:

	3 Months	5 Months
FVC	2.40 L (67%)	2.06 L (59%)
FEV1	1.99 L (72%)	0.86 L (31%)
TLC	3.42 L (70%)	3.32 L (68%)

At 7 months she was able to walk only a block, and exam revealed rales at both lung bases. Chest radiography revealed normal lung fields. A course of antithymocyte serum was administered for chronic rejection/bronchiolitis obliterans.

Her clinical course stabilized during the following year. Occasional periods of increased dyspnea on exertion were associated with increased production of discolored sputum, and these episodes generally responded to oral antibiotics. Her evaluation at 1 year after transplant included right heart catheterization, which revealed pulmonary artery pressure of 34/18, mean = 20 mm Hg.

Twenty-three months after transplantation she noted a subacute decline in her functional capacity and worse dyspnea. Two cavities were observed on chest radiography in the right upper lobe and bronchoscopic sampling confirmed aspergillus infection. The cavities enlarged daily despite amphotericin and then itraconazole therapy for 3 weeks, when massive hemoptysis occurred and resuscitation was not successful. Postmortem examination confirmed severe bronchiolitis obliterans and two 3-cm cavities in the right upper lobe, with arteriocavitary and bronchial hemorrhage.

FINAL DIAGNOSES

Bronchiolitis obliterans complicating heart–lung transplantation; fatal massive hemoptysis from progressive invasive aspergillus.

DISCUSSION

Bronchiolitis obliterans was recognized as the major long-term complication of heart–lung transplantation in the late 1980s. The incidence of this catastrophic complication varies among transplant centers but has occurred in the majority of patients in some large studies. Although its onset has generally occurred years after transplantation, it can occur early, within a few months of transplantation, as unfortunately was the case in the patient presented here. As single lung transplantation was introduced in the early 1990s bronchiolitis appeared to be a rare complication, but with larger experience it appears that the incidence of bronchiolitis as a complication of lung transplant is in the range 20–25% regardless of the specific procedure, that is, single lung, both lungs, or heart–lung.

The pathogenetic mechanisms of bronchiolitis obliterans are poorly understood, although it is generally considered to be a manifestation of chronic rejection. Some studies suggest an association of bronchiolitis with recurrent episodes of rejection, or with symptomatic cytomegalovirus infection. It is not known whether such events actually trigger bronchiolitis or whether they are simply markers of patients at risk.

Therapy of patients with bronchiolitis obliterans complicating lung transplantation is controversial and unproven. A general approach has been to increase the immunosuppression, but corticosteroids, cyclosporin, or imuran have not been successful. Treatment with antilymphocyte preparations, such as that given in this patient, may be associated with stabilization of the process in a significant proportion of patients. Whereas the decline in pulmonary function related to acute rejection is reversible, the pathophysiologic dysfunction caused by bronchiolitis is not reversible and is usually progressive. Bronchiolitis obliterans is the most significant long-term complication of lung transplantation procedures and justifies intensified research efforts to understand pathogenesis and devise new preventive or therapeutic strategies.

LATE COMPLICATIONS AFTER HEART–LUNG TRANSPLANTATION

Some complications are the following:

Acute lung rejection
Acute heart rejection
Airway anastomotic dehiscence/stenosis
Chronic rejection/bronchiolitis obliterans
Infection

Aspergillus Infection in Lung Transplant Patients

Recipients of lung transplants appear to be at greater risk of infection than recipients of other solid-organ transplants. Lung recipients are at increased risk for organisms from all classifications, including bacterial, viral, and fungal. Infections with fungi, especially aspergillus, may be especially difficult to manage successfully, as is demonstrated in this patient. Aspergillus has a special proclivity to invade vessels, which can lead to the catastrophic outcome of massive hemoptysis, as took the life of this patient. Fungal infections in either the airway or vascular anastomoses have been major problems in the perioperative period, which has led to the use of antifungal prophylactic regimens during the perioperative period in many centers. Although the recent development of oral antifungal agents with relatively low toxicity has been a significant advance, the efficacy of these agents against aspergillus is generally inadequate, and better agents are greatly needed.

BIBLIOGRAPHY

DUMMER JS, MONTERO CG, GRIFFITH BP, HARDESTY RL, PARADIS IL, HO M. Infections in heart–lung transplant recipients. *Transplantation* 1986;41:725–729.

DUMMER JS. Infectious complications following heart–lung transplantation—the Pittsburgh experience. In *Lung & Heart–Lung Transplantation.* 1991. ed V. Gallucci, U. Livi, G. Foggian, A. Mazzu (Pichon Nuova Libraria; Padua) p. 135–147.

HORVATH J, DUMMER SJ, LOYD JE, WALKER B, MERRILL WH, FRIST WH. Infection in the transplanted and native lung after single lung transplantation. *Chest* in press.

PARADIS IL, DUNCAN SR, DAUBER JH, COSTANTINO JP, SIMILO S, YOUSEM SA, HARDESTY RL, GRIFFITH BP. Effect of augmented immunosuppression on human chronic lung allograft rejection. *Am Rev Resp Dis* 146:1213–1215, 1992.

SCOTT JP, HIGENBOTTAM TW, SHARPLES L, CLELLAND CA, SMYTH RL, STEWART S, WALLWORK, J. Risk factors for obliterative bronchiolitis in heart-lung transplant recipients. *Transplantation* 1991;51:813–817.

YOUSEM SA, DAUBER JA, KEENAN R, PARADIS IL, ZEEVI A, GRIFFITH BP. Does histologic acute rejection in lung allografts predict the development of bronchiolitis obliterans. *Transplantation* 1991;52:306–309.

15

Photopheresis for Chronic Rejection in Lung Transplantation

*B.S. Slovis, L.E. King, Jr., L. Lawrence,
J.R. Stewart, and J.E. Loyd*

CASE 1

History

A 21-year-old female received a right single lung transplant on June 21, 1991, for pulmonary hypertension related to a congenital ventriculoseptal defect (VSD). Despite repair of her VSD at age 4, she developed progressive pulmonary hypertension in her late teens and was subsequently bedbound by right heart failure. She initially responded to calcium antagonist therapy for pulmonary vasodilation, but the functional improvement lasted less than a year. At the time of transplantation, she had been returned to a chair-to-bed existence. Right and left heart catheterization performed 1 year prior to transplant revealed pulmonary hypertension that was suprasystemic; pulmonary artery (PA) pressure was 150/80 mm Hg, mean = 115 mm Hg, and pulmonary artery wedge pressure was 10 mm Hg. Systemic blood pressure was 100/60 mm Hg and cardiac output was 3.3 L/min. Her serology for cytomegalovirus (CMV) was positive and the donor was CMV negative. She had never smoked and had no other significant past medical history.

Hospital Course

The patient received a cadaveric single lung transplant on June 21, 1991, with an end-to-end anastomosis and omental wrap. Initial standard immunosuppressive therapy included azathioprine, cyclosporine, prednisone, and antithymocyte serum for 14 days. Reimplantation pulmonary edema led to delayed weaning from repeat bronchoscopy, once again her anastomosis was well healed and widely patent. Thoracoscopic lung biopsy confirmed the diagnosis of BOOP. A planned 14-day course of antithymocyte serum was discontinued after 7 days due to an urticarial rash. At that time she had antiheterophil antibodies positive to rabbit, and her circulating lymphocyte count had not fallen after beginning Anti-thymocyte Serum (ATS). Her symptoms progressed further and her function declined. ATS therapy was judged to have been ineffective and on September 5, 1992 OKT3 therapy was begun with the goal to arrest the progression of bronchiolitis. Fifteen minutes after beginning the infusion, she became tachycardic, hypoxic, and hypotensive, requiring emergent intubation and pharmacologic hemodynamic support. Broad-spectrum antibiotics were initiated, but cultures remained negative and it was felt that this clinical syndrome was related to a massive cytokine release syndrome from OKT3 infusion. She required prolonged mechanical ventilation but was eventually weaned to a Bipap mask and on October 7, 1992 she was discharged home with supplemental oxygen at 4 L/min.

On October 27, 1992, follow-up pulmonary function testing revealed a further decline in her FEV1 to 940 cc. Based on reports of successful treatment of acute rejection in heart transplant recipients, she was offered photopheresis as an experimental rescue therapy for her bronchiolitis/chronic rejection. Photopheresis was initiated on November 11, 1992 according to the following protocol. On two consecutive days each month, 2 h after oral administration of 8-methoxypsoralen (Psoralen), 0.5 mg/kg, the patient receives mechanical ventilation. In addition, her postoperative course was complicated by CMV infection and an episode of acute rejection which responded to high-dose steroids. She was discharged July 31, 1991 on 2 L oxygen by nasal cannula with a postoperative forced expiratory volume at first second (FEV1) of 1.56 L.

She improved and did very well during the next year and did not require supplemental oxygen. She returned to college and was married 11 months after her transplant. Shortly before her annual evaluation in June 1992, she began to experience gradually increasing dyspnea on exertion. At that time her FEV1 was stable at 2.03 L, but bronchoscopy with transbronchial biopsy revealed stenosis of her anastomosis and moderate rejection, grade 2. She was admitted for YAG-laser excision of her stenosis on July 22, 1992 with symptoms of increasing dyspnea and a dry cough. In the interval, her FEV1 had declined to 1.60 L. Repeat transbronchial biopsy confirmed the diagnosis of moderate rejection. Resting room air oxygen saturations were 89% to 92% and she was discharged on home oxygen on July 26, 1992. On July 27, 1992 she was readmitted with a pseudomonas pneumonia in her native lung, which responded promptly to I.V. antibiotics. Repeat bronchoscopy demonstrated good healing of her anastomosis, which was widely patent. Her immunosuppressive regimen on discharge was cylosporine 100 mg bid, azathioprine 125 mg qd, and prednisone 20 mg qd.

Her dyspnea continued to worsen and she was readmitted on August 24, 1992, after an outside transbronchial biopsy revealed bronchiolitis obliterans with organizing pneumonia (BOOP). At discontinuous leukapheresis with exposure of the leukocytes to ultraviolet A light followed by reinfusion. Each photopheresis session takes approximately 3.5 h. She has received monthly photopheresis since that time. Her pulmonary function tests have improved and her FEV1 is stable at 1.3 L in 18 months of follow-up. Figure 15-1 is a graph of the change in her FEV1 with time since her transplant. She remains on cyclosporine and azathioprine and has gradually been weaned to 10 mg of prednisone a day without exacerbation of symptoms. She has substantial functional limitations and requires supplemental oxygen but has been stable nearly 2 years since beginning photopheresis.

CASE 2: FRANK HAYNIE

A 50-year-old white male received a right single lung transplant December 7, 1991 for severe emphysema. He had smoked cigarettes until age 40 when he was told he had emphysema. In his late forties, he had developed progressive exertional limitation. He was only able to walk 25 yards and had developed dyspnea at rest. He had transiently required mechanical ventilation for respiratory failure on one occasion. Pulmonary function testing prior to transplantation revealed a forced vital capacity (FVC) of 3.5 L and a forced expiratory volume in the first second (FEV1) of 0.5 L.

On December 7, 1991 he received a single lung cadaveric transplant. The perioperative period for transplantation was uncomplicated and he left hospital after 17 days. Pulmonary function testing improved substantially until on April 7, 1992 his FVC was 4.32 L and his FEV1 was 2.43 L. A few months later, June 5, 1992, when his spirometry

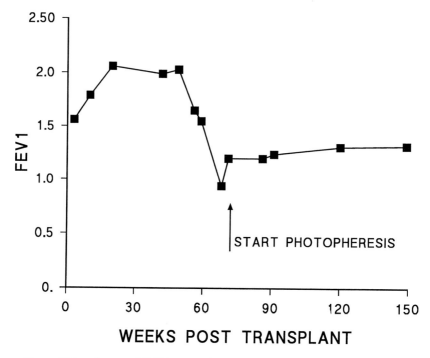

Figure 15-1. Change of FEV1 versus time since transplant.

declined slightly, bronchoscopy was performed and transbronchial biopsies were normal. A perfusion scan on August 24, 1992 revealed that 87% of pulmonary blood flow went to the right transplanted lung, but there was a new small perfusion defect. Pulmonary arteriography was normal, but bronchoscopy revealed mild rejection on biopsy.

He continued to demonstrate a progressive decline in his FEV1 and on March 11, 1993 was diagnosed with BOOP on open lung biopsy. Due to lack of response to increased doses of prednisone and worsening renal function with increased doses of cyclosporine, he was offered photopheresis as an experimental therapy. He began photopheresis on March 18, 1993 according to the protocol described in the previous case. Since that time he has had no further exacerbations of rejection and his FEV1 has remained stable in 15 months of follow-up.

Discussion

Photopheresis is a technique for immunomodulation of cell-mediated immunity. It was first described as a successful treatment of cutaneous T-cell lymphoma (CTCL) by Edelson et al. in 1987 [1]. It is now an accepted and sometimes first-line therapy for this disease. Its use has expanded to include treatment of some autoimmune diseases such as scleroderma, pemphigus vulgaris, and juvenile dermatomyositis [2, 3]. More recently, promising clinical trials have been conducted in rheumatoid arthritis, multiple sclerosis, insulin-dependent diabetes mellitus, and AIDS-related complex [2].

Based on results from studies in skin allograft rejection in mice [4], Costanzo-Norton and colleagues successfully employed photopheresis as an experimental rescue therapy for acute rejection following heart transplant [5]. They performed a preliminary randomized trial of photopheresis versus corticosteroids in 16 patients with acute heart transplant rejection. The results suggested that photopheresis may be as effective as corticosteroids in the treatment of acute rejection. Importantly, this and other studies have not shown any significant toxicities or side effects of photopheresis. Photopheresis appears to have no effect on normal-cell-mediated immune function and has allowed reductions in dosage of immunosuppressive drugs in some patients being treated for autoimmune disease [2, 6].

The mechanism of action of photopheresis is not fully understood although several probable mechanisms have been identified. Psoralen is taken up by leukocytes and remains inactive until exposed to ultraviolet A radiation. Activated psoralen leads to cross-linking of DNA, which prevents further cell proliferation. Damaged cells are then rapidly destroyed. This process seems to affect activated mononuclear cells preferentially. The destruction of activated T cells is not thought to be the primary mechanism of immunomodulation, however. Animal models of T-cell-mediated autoimmune disease and transplant rejection suggest a vaccination effect of photomodulated cells against the pathogenic T-cell clones [7]. Specifically, suppressor T cells seem to develop in response to the phototreated cells.

Although the precise mode of action of photopheresis is incompletely understood, its preliminary efficacy in the treatment of cell-mediated immune disease and response to solid organ transplant combined with its apparent safety and lack of significant side effects make it a promising avenue for future research and clinical trials. To our knowledge, these are the first lung transplant recipients to undergo photopheresis for BOOP. After 15 and 18 months of therapy, their pulmonary function remains stable. The optimal interval and duration of photopheresis therapy for BOOP following lung transplant is unknown. Given the absence of demonstrated toxicity we have elected to continue monthly treatments indefinitely as long as their pulmonary function does not decline.

REFERENCES

1. Edelson R, Berger C, Gasparro F et al. Treatment of cutaneous T-cell lymphoma by extracorporeal photochemotherapy. Preliminary results. *N Engl J Med* 1987;316:297–303.
2. Rook AH, Cohen JH, Lessin SR, Vowels BR. Therapeutic applications of photopheresis. *Derm Clin* 1993;11:339–347.
3. DeWilde A, DiSpaltro F, Geller A et al. Extracorporeal photochemotherapy as adjunctive treatment in juvenile dermatomyositis: A case report. *Arch Dermatol* 1992;128:1656–1657.
4. Perez MI, Edelson RL, Laroche L, Berger C. Inhibition of antiskin allograft immunity by infusions with syngeneic photoinactivated effector lymphocytes. *J Invest Dermatol* 1989;92:669–676.
5. Costanzo-Nordin MR, Hubbell EA, O'Sullivan EJ et al. Photopheresis versus corticosteroids in the therapy of heart transplant rejection. Preliminary clinical report. *Circulation* 1992;86(Suppl. 5):II242–II250.
6. Vowels BR, Berkson M, Cohen J et al. Extracorporeal photopheresis (ExP) does not suppress T or B cell responses to recall or novel antigens (Abstract). *J Invest Dermatol* 1992;98:686–692.
7. Khavari PA, Edelson RL, Lider O et al. Specific vaccination against photoinactivated cloned T cells (Abstract). *Clin Res* 1991;36:662A.

16

Pancytopenia Following Liver Transplantation for Fulminant Hepatic Failure in a Young Male

Anne T. Thomas and Ellen B. Hunter

CASE PRESENTATION

History of the Present Illness

The patient is a 14-year-old male who noted the onset of nausea, vomiting, and malaise on May 1, 1991. Two days later, the patient was seen in his pediatrician's office and noted to be jaundiced. Laboratory studies performed included a serum bilirubin, which was 6.5 mg/dl, and an amino-leuyl transferase (ALT) of 2601 IU/L. The patient was admitted with the presumptive diagnosis of hepatitis and dehydration. Further studies included hepatitis A, B, and C serologies, which were negative. A mono spot test was nonreactive. The patient denied previous blood transfusion, I.V. drug use, or acetaminophen intake. Three months prior to the onset of this illness, the patient was stuck in the thigh by a straight pin by a schoolmate. None of the schoolmates had known hepatitis.

During the hospitalization, the patient was rehydrated and serial laboratory tests were obtained. On May 8, 1991 a bilirubin was 14.3 mg/dl with an ALT of 2057 IU/L. The patient's oral intake improved and he was discharged on May 10, 1991 with close follow-up as an outpatient. Three days later, the patient was readmitted for worsening jaundice (bilirubin 30.2 mg/dl) and coagulopathy with a prothrombin time of 20 s. Because of the worsening liver tests, the patient was transferred to the pediatric gastroenterology service at Vanderbilt University for further evaluation and management. The patient's past medical history was remarkable for Salmonella gastroenteritis as a toddler and abdominal pain secondary to gastritis in 1986. The patient had no history of previous surgery and was presently on no medications including acetaminophen.

Physical Examination

Examination presented the following: Blood pressure 97/52 mm Hg, pulse 67/min, temperature 99.6 °F, and respiratory rate 32/min. Examination of the skin revealed icterus without spider angiomata. The examination of the head and neck revealed scleral icterus without Kayser–Fleischer rings. The orophyarnx was benign. There was no thyromegaly or adenopathy. The lungs were clear and the cardiovascular examination was within normal limits. The abdominal examination revealed normal bowel sounds with a palpable liver edge 1 cm below the right costal margin. There was mild right upper quadrant tenderness with deep inspiration. Splenomegaly and ascites were not present. There was no peripheral edema. Neurologic examination was intact and there was no asterixis.

Laboratory Evaluation

The laboratory tests presented the following

		Normal Range
WBC	3500/mm^3	4–11,000
Hematocrit	42%	42–50
Platelet count	199,000/mm^3	150–400,000
Bilirubin	29.4 mg/dl	0.2–1.2
AST	2260 IU/L	4–40
ALT	2180 IU/L	4–40
Albumin	3.7 g/dl	3.5–5
Alk. phos.	223 IU/L	50–375
PT	26 s (INR 4.5)	10–13
APTT	53 s	25–40
Fibrinogen	105 mg/dl	190–400
Sodium	139 mEq/L	135–145
Potassium	4.1 mEq/L	3.5–5
Chloride	95 mEq/L	95–105
CO$_2$	36 mmol/L	18–27
Glucose	103 mg/dl	70–110
BUN	7 mg/dl	5–25

| Creatinine | 0.6 mg/dl | 0–1.2 |
| Ammonia | 44µmol/L | 11–35 |

Hospital Course

The patient was admitted with the diagnosis of acute hepatitis with severe hepatic impairment. Treatment with lactulose, neomycin, parenteral vitamin K supplementation, histamine-2 antagonist, and low-protein diet was instituted. Etiologies for acute hepatitis including hepatitis A, B, C, Wilson's disease, alpha 1-antitrypsin deficiency, hemochromatosis, and autoimmune hepatitis were excluded. Serial laboratory studies revealed worsening liver tests with a prolonged prothrombin time of 40 s, (INR 9.7) and a serum bilirubin of 30.9 mg/dl. Because of the probability of further deterioration, the patient was evaluated for liver transplantation and placed on the waiting list. On May 18, 1991, the patient developed lethargy without asterixis (stage 1 encephalopathy) which progressed over the next 2 days to a comatose state (stage 4 encephalopathy.) The patient's severe coagulopathy was partially corrected with fresh frozen plasma and cryoprecipitate. Because of the patient's deteriorating mental status, he was intubated, given intravenous mannitol, and an intracranial pressure monitor was placed. The initial intracerebral pressure was normal at 7 mm Hg. The patient required a constant glucose infusion for hypoglycemia.

Four days after being placed on the transplant waiting list an ABO compatible (blood type O positive) donor was identified for this type AB positive recipient. The donor organ was cytomegalovirus (CMV) positive by serology and the patient was negative. During the anhepatic phase of the transplant operation, the intracranial pressure reached 21 mm Hg which was treated with I.V. mannitol. Nonirradiated blood products were used intraoperatively. Postoperatively the patient initially did well with excellent allograft function. The patient was extubated 2 days postoperatively and his mental status cleared. Immunosuppression was administered as cyclosporine 100 mg I.V. over 24 h, azathioprine 75 mg I.V. daily, and methylprednisolone 50 mg I.V. qid. The patient's posttransplant course was complicated by rejection, which required methylprednisolone boluses and 5 days of OKT3 antilymphocyte monoclonal antibody beginning on postoperative day 8. He also received anti-CMV immunoglobulin and empiric gancyclovir. On the third postoperavite day the patient's blood counts decreased to WBC 1700/mm^3 with 81% polys, 8% atypical lymphocytes, 10% monocytes, and 1% eosinophils; hematocrit 31%, and platelet count 52,000/mm3. Myelosuppressive medications including azathioprine were discontinued. He also developed a positive direct Coombs' test with anti-A eluted from his red cells. His pancytopenia continued to worsen and a bone marrow aspiration and biopsy performed on postoperative day 13 revealed aplasia. Cultures of the marrow were negative.

His white blood cell count remained below $500/mm^3$ for 6 days. He did not experience any serious infections but received antibiotics for neutropenic fevers. The patient's blood counts were supported with ir-radiated blood products (type O red cells), erythropoietin, and escalat-ing doses of recombinant granulocyte-colony stimulating factor (G-CSF). Because of the possibility of non-A, non-B viral hepatitis-associated aplastic anemia, the patient was treated with an antiviral agent, riba-virin, experimental for this indication, intravenously for 10 days. His was given two 225-mg boluses of methylprednisolone in addition to his regular cyclosporine and 30 mg prednisone per day. A random skin biopsy did not show any histologic change suggestive of graft-versus-host disease. Peripheral lymphocyte typing studies were identical to his pretransplant phenotype. Parvovirus B19 studies by serology and poly-merase chain reaction were negative. The patient's blood counts slowly increased and a follow-up bone marrow examination on postoperative day 29 revealed some improvement in cellularity compared to the orig-inal study. His positive direct Coombs' test persisted throughout his hospitalization and anti-B was identified transiently as well as the per-sistent anti-A which peaked at a titre of 1:16. On the day of discharge, 38 days posttransplant, the patient's blood counts were improved with a WBC of $11,100/mm^3$, hematocrit 29%, and platelet count of 56,000/mm^3.

Three months posttransplant, the patient's blood counts decreased with a WBC of $3400/mm^3$, hematocrit 29.7%, and platelet count of $66,000/mm^3$. The patient had experienced an antecedent viral syn-drome. Another course of ribavirin was administered for 10 days with-out benefit and, in fact, was associated with mild hemolysis. Additional blood products were required as well as G-CSF and increased oral pred-nisone. Later, a report positive for CMV IgM was received. A gradual rise in his blood counts ensued and he remains well.

DISCUSSION OF THE DIFFERENTIAL DIAGNOSIS

The case presented is that of pancytopenia developing after liver trans-plantation in a young male with fulminant hepatic failure and coma from non-A, non-B, non-C hepatitis. Other pertinent information in his case is his CMV negative status while his liver graft was CMV positive. The differential diagnosis of pancytopenia is quite extensive and this case presents several plausible explanations.

Aplastic anemia is of prime consideration and has many causes or associated conditions. Approximately half of the cases are associated with drug reactions [1]. Although most patients with drug-associated aplastic anemia do not respond to withdrawal of the offending drug, some cases may improve. Drugs such as azathioprine and various antibiotics are frequently implicated in pancytopenia. His azathioprine, gancyclovir, and vancomycin were stopped by the third postoperative day and all other medicines were kept to an absolute minimum. Given the very short period of time he was exposed to these medicines (1 day and 2 days) prior to his severe pancytopenia, their likelihood as etiologic agents is low.

Infectious causes were screened with viral, fungal, and bacterial cultures of the marrow, which were all negative. Hepatitis has a well-known association with pancytopenia and aplastic anemia, particularly so-called non-A, non-B, non-C virus(es) and occasionally hepatitis B virus. There is no specific test or study to verify the hepatitis association, and this is a diagnosis of exclusion.

In this special case, graft-versus-host disease induced by passenger lymphocytes in the new liver or by lymphocytes in the many blood products he received must be considered as well. Graft-versus-host-disease (GVHD) from T lymphocytes transplanted with the liver or received with a blood transfusion may cause depressed marrow function and carries a high mortality rate in immunosuppressed patients [2]. Typing of his peripheral lymphocytes indicated that he was maintaining his original HLA typing pattern and not developing an immune system chimera, evidence against engraftment of any exogenous T lymphocytes. A random skin biopsy was not consistent with GVHD either. However, the B lymphocytes passively transported with the blood type O positive liver graft into his type AB positive body began synthesizing measurable and clinically significant levels of IgG anti-A and anti-B blood group antibodies. Erythrophagocytosis was noted in his marrow smears and his hematocrit was falling without evidence of bleeding; therefore, his postoperative RBC transfusions were changed to type O positive cells. However, the very earliest bone marrow progenitor cells do not express A or B antigens on their surface. Although this particular graft-versus-host phenomenon complicated his course, it cannot be implicated as a cause of his pancytopenia.

Infections with other marrow-suppressing viruses such as parvovirus B19 and particularly cytomegalovirus are of serious concern in a transplant patient given his CMV-positive liver graft and probable CMV positive blood products (unscreened because his graft was seropositive). Viral studies including polymerase chain reaction tests for parvovirus B19 and hepatitis C RNA were negative. He received anti-CMV enriched immunoglobulin after transplant and every 2 weeks thereafter for 6 weeks. At no time during his hospital course did he have any positive cultures or positive serologies for acute CMV infection. However, after discharge, his recovery of marrow function suffered a setback associated with a viral syndrome and the appearance of anti-CMV IgM.

With normal blood counts at the onset of his illness, one is much less likely to place a primary marrow disease such as leukemia or myelodysplasia, or a metastatic neoplasm near the top of the list. It also appeared a bit early posttransplantation, making an immunosuppression-related lymphoma with marrow invasion an unlikely candidate.

In any patient with pancytopenia without obvious cause, a bone marrow examination is necessary. Figure 16-1 shows a markedly hypocel-

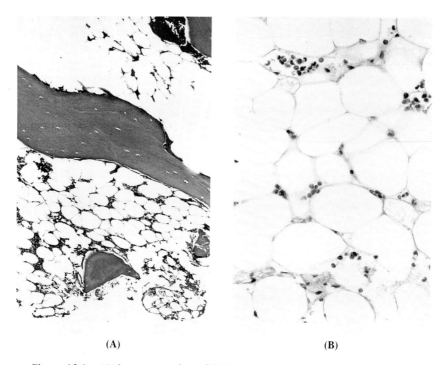

(A)   (B)

Figure 16-1. (*A*) Low-power view of PAS stain of biopsy showing marked hypocellularity; (*B*) reveals very few normal marrow elements at higher magnification diagnostic of severe aplastic anemia.

lular marrow with very few normal marrow elements, no tumor or granulomata present, diagnostic of severe aplastic anemia.

DIAGNOSIS

The diagnosis was non-A, non-B, non-C hepatitis-associated aplastic anemia.

DISCUSSION

Since the first reported association of hepatitis and aplastic anemia in 1955 many characteristic features have been described, but an etiologic agent(s) has yet to be elucidated [3]. This particular case is typical in many ways. Patients usually develop aplasia within 1 month of the onset of hepatitis, are more often male, and frequently less than 20 years old. Although most patients are actually experiencing an improvement in their hepatitis when they develop aplastic anemia, a strikingly increased incidence (28%) of aplasia has been noted in fulminant hepatic failure of uncertain etiology, requiring liver transplantation as in this young man's case. It has been proposed that a yet-to-be-discovered hepatitis F virus is responsible for both processes [4].

In American and European series of aplastic anemia, hepatitis precedes the pancytopenia in 2–5% of cases. However, in the Orient that proportion is much higher at approximately 10%. The overall incidence of aplasia in the Far East is greater and rivals that of acute myelogenous leukemia, whereas in the United States, acute leukemia is 10 times more common than aplastic anemia. Oriental immigrants living in the United States develop aplastic anemia at the U.S. rate, suggesting an environmental factor. Although hepatitis may be a relatively infrequent cause of aplastic anemia, the cases are quite remarkable for their severity and high mortality rates exceeding 85% [5].

Initially, evidence for a putative virus was lacking, as few serologic tests were available. Later data revealed a small number of aplastics with antibodies, suggesting hepatitis B infection, and even some case reports of hepatitis A. However, the majority were serologically negative or non-A, non-B. Until sensitive and specific tests (including reverse transcriptase-polymerase chain reaction) for hepatitis C virus RNA became available, it was the primary suspect in the search for the villain. Recent studies have cast grave doubts on this theory as the frequency of positive tests for hepatitis C in aplastic patients is not higher than that observed in the control population or the frequency of hepatitis C was found to be most dependent on the number of transfusions the patient received prior to testing and not on the purported etiology of the aplasia [6, 7].

The pathophysiology of the aplasia is still poorly understood. Direct infection of marrow elements has been shown for non-A, non-B virus in chimpanzees. The virus was most likely what is now recognized as hepatitis C although testing was not available at that time. Hepatitis A and B viruses have also been shown to inhibit the in vitro growth of pluripotential progenitor cells and committed stem cells. However, the serologic evidence does not support any of these viruses as the primary culprit [8].

There is strong evidence to suggest an autoimmune reactive response directed against the marrow. Flow cytometry studies have revealed an immune deficiency particularly in children developing aplastic anemia after hepatitis that has not been typical of the idiopathic cases [9]. Some groups have reported increases in activated suppressor T lymphocytes (and increases in gamma interferon) while others have found increased percentages of these cells, but marked overall depression in the total numbers of lymphocytes did not manifest as an absolute rise in activated suppressor cells [10]. Elevated levels of granulocyte–macrophage colony stimulating factor (GM-CSF), a product of activated T lymphocytes, were found in aplastic patients and might be associated with a response to immunosuppressive therapy [11]. Depressed T lymphocyte helper:suppressor ratios have also been observed to ratios less than 1.0 and even frequently 0.5. A T-cell line was developed from a patient with hepatitis-associated aplastic anemia that inhibited erythroid, granulocyte, and monocyte colony formation in vitro, leading the investigators to speculate that a viral infection activated a specific population of suppressor T lymphocytes, which inhibited hematopoiesis [12]. Still, the specific sequence of events leading to this devastating complication of hepatitis eludes us.

Therapeutic Approach

Supportive care measures are critical to patient management from the moment of diagnosis throughout therapy. Transfusion of red blood cells and platelets should be instituted as needed with consideration of leukopoor products (typically by filter) from the outset in the hope of delaying or decreasing the likelihood of anti-HLA antibody development. This will diminish febrile transfusion reactions and delay (or prevent) platelet refractoriness and resistance to bone marrow engraftment. CMV negative products are indicated if the patient's serology studies are negative especially for those patients for whom bone marrow transplant is planned. Treatment of infections is usually empiric at the onset of fever during neutropenic periods. Broad-spectrum antibiotics covering the more rapidly fatal gram negative infections as well as the more likely (if an indwelling catheter is in place) gram positive organisms are begun immediately prior to receipt of microbiologic reports. Antifungal agents need to be considered early if fever persists on broad-spectrum coverage [13].

Bone marrow transplantation is the treatment of choice for severe aplastic anemia in patients less than 50 years old with an HLA-matched sibling donor. In children less than 10 years old without a matched sibling donor, an aggressive search for an unrelated HLA-matched volunteer donor is indicated as results from a full phenotypic match will rival those from HLA-matched siblings. Graft survival seems to be inversely related to the number of pretransplant transfusions the patient receives. Therefore, in severe cases the transplant should proceed as soon as a donor can be found. Cell dose is related to engraftment since those receiving 3.0×10^8 cells per kilogram or more are less likely to reject the transplant. Cyclosporine posttransplant has also reduced graft rejection and is continued for at least 1 year [13]. Patients who are transplanted successfully have a lower likelihood of late sequelae such as paroxysmal nocturnal hemoglobinuria, myelodysplasia, and acute leukemia than those treated with immunosuppression alone [14, 15].

Medical management of aplastic anemia consists of empiric immunosuppression to allow the marrow to recover function. Therapeutic options consist mainly of steroids, antilymphocyte globulin, and cyclosporine. Other monoclonal antilymphocyte antibodies, androgenic steroids, and splenectomy have been tried with varying success.

Antilymphocyte globulin (ALG) can produce remissions in 35–65% of patients with effectiveness dependent on the initial severity. Those with neutrophil counts less than 0.2×10^9/L, particularly if they are infected, will have remission rates at the lower end of the range. Young children <6 years old respond poorly to ALG treatment, but adults over 25 do as well with immunosuppressive therapy as comparable bone marrow transplant candidates. The mechanism of action of these antibodies grown against human lymphocytes is not entirely clear. They reduce the number of circulating lymphocytes but also may have stimulatory effects on other hematopoietic elements producing cytokines or enhance responsiveness to growth factors. The main side effects include fever and chills, rash, and thrombocytopenia. Serious events such as fluid retention, anaphylaxis, hypertension, and seizures have been reported. Serum sickness can occur approximately 7–10 days after therapy, especially if corticosteroids are not given concomitantly. Response is not immediate but typically occurs in 6–12 weeks [16]. Approximately one-third of patients that do not respond to ALG initially may improve with a second course [13].

Corticosteroids have been used for years. The dose range required for any benefits produces some prohibitive side effects including increased risk for infection, hypertension, and marked glucose interance. In one study where very high-dose steroids (20 mg methylprednisolone/kg and taper) plus antithymocyte globulin and oxymetholone were compared to lower-dose steroids (0.5 mg/kg methylprednisolone) plus antithymocyte globulin and oxymetholone, there were no significant differences in outcome or toxicity [17].

Cyclosporine A (CsA) is effective in inducing responses in severe aplastic anemia at about the same rate as ALG. One recent study comparing CsA alone with antithymocyte globulin (ATG) with prednisone and subsequent crossover treatment did not show a significant difference in survival between the groups. At 12 months the actuarial survival was 70% in the CsA group and 64% in the ATG group. Infections were observed more often and were more often lethal in the ATG and prednisone group. Cyclosporine shows promise as an effective therapy in those for whom bone marrow transplantation is not feasible or indicated [18].

Other treatment regimens including intravenous immunoglobulin [19], various hematopoietic growth factors such as IL-3, granulocyte colony-stimulating factor [20], granulocyte-macrophage colony-stimulating factor, and acycloguanosine [21] have been tried with some reported successes.

The long-term prognosis for these patients depends on the severity of the initial pancytopenia and treatment regimen employed. Bone marrow transplantation (BMT) not only produces the highest early survival in the best cases (80%) but is also essentially free of the continuing incidence of other serious marrow complications such as paroxysmal nocturnal hemoglobinuria, myelodysplasia, acute leukemia, and recurrence of aplasia seen in nongrafted patients. However, BMT does carry its own set of potential future problems such as a 10% risk of chronic graft-versus-host disease, and risks of the conditioning regimen (sterilization, secondary malignancy, and pulmonary, endocrine, and other chronic ailments.) Actuarial survival curves in nongrafted patient populations may not plateau for 6–12 years of follow-up. In the French aplastic anemia cooperative study of patients alive 5 years after diagnosis, at 10 years postdiagnosis (70% evaluable subjects remaining), most had normal blood counts despite abnormal marrow stem cell concentrations and had an excellent quality of life [15]. A Swiss study reported a continuously increasing risk of late hematologic complications of severe aplastic anemia in nongrafted patients that reached 57% at 8 years [14]. Treatment of late complications remains wholly inadequate at this time.

SUMMARY

This young man developed aplastic anemia, a devastating complication of fulminant hepatic failure from non-A, non-B, non-C hepatitis that required liver transplantation. His marrow has appeared to respond to early immunosuppressive therapy given primarily for his liver graft and he maintains an excellent quality of life 2 years following his transplant with blood counts of WBC $9200/mm^2$, hematocrit 34.6%, and platelet count of $131,000/mm^3$. However, he does remain at risk for late hematologic sequelae.

ACKNOWLEDGMENTS

Elizabeth Caldwell, M.D. kindly provided the photomicrographs. Sanford B. Krantz, M.D. gave many thoughtful suggestions and comments for which we are grateful.

REFERENCES

1. Young NS. The pathogenesis and pathophysiology of aplastic anemia. In: Hoffman R, Berz, Jr. EJ, Shattil SJ, Fourie B, Cohen T, ed. *Hematology: Basic Principles & Practice*. New York: Churchill Livingstone, 1991: p. 122–160.
2. Anderson KC, Goodnough LT, Sayers M et al. Variation in blood component irradiation practice: Implications for prevention of transfusion-associated graft-versus-host disease. *Blood* 1991;77:2096–2102.
3. Hagler L, Pastore RA, Bergin JJ, Wrensch MR. Aplastic anemia following viral hepatitis: Report of two fatal cases and literature review. *Medicine* 1975;54:139–164.
4. Hibbs JR, Frickhofen N, Rosenfeld SJ et al. Aplastic anemia and viral hepatitis non-A, non-B, non-C? *J Am Med Assoc* 1992;267:2051–2054.
5. Young NS. Flaviviruses and bone marrow failure. *J Am Med Assoc* 1990;263:3065–3068.
6. Pol S, Driss F, Devergie A et al. Is hepatitis C virus involved in hepatitis-associated aplastic anemia? *Ann Intern Med* 1990;113:435–437.

7. Wright TL, Hsu H, Donegan E et al. Hepatitis C virus not found in fulminant non-A, non-B hepatitis. *Ann Intern Med* 1991;115:111–112.
8. Zeldis JB, Beonder PJ, Hellings JA, Steinberg H. Inhibition of human hemopoiesis by non-A, non-B hepatitis virus. *J Med Virol* 1989;27:34–38.
9. Foon KA, Mitsuyasu RT, Schroff RW et al. Immunologic defects in young male patients with hepatitis-associated aplastic anemia. *Ann Intern Med* 1984;100:657–662.
10. Kojima S, Matsuyama K, Kodera Y, Okada J. Circulating activated suppressor T lymphocytes in hepatitis-associated aplastic anemia. *Br J Haematol* 1989;71:147–151.
11. Schrezenmeier H, Raghavachar A, Heimpel H. Granulocyte-macrophage colony stimulating factor in the sera of patients with aplastic anemia. *Clin Invest* 1993;71:102–108.
12. Herrman F, Griffin JD, Meuer SG, Zum Bushenfelder KM. Establishment of an interleukin-2 dependent T cell line derived from a patient with severe aplastic anemia, which inhibits in vitro hematopoiesis. *J Immunol* 1986;136:1629–1634.
13. Gordon-Smith EC. Acquired aplastic anemia. In: *Hematology: Basic Principles & Practice*. New York: Churchill Livingstone, 1991:160–172.
14. Tichelli A, Gratwohl A, Wursch A, Nissen C, Speck B. Late haematological complications in severe aplastic anemia. *Br J Haematol* 1988;69:413–418.
15. Najean Y, Haguenauer O. Long-term (5 to 20 years) evolution of non-grafted aplastic anemias. *Blood* 1990;76:2222–2228.
16. Champlin R, Ho W, Gale RP. Antithymocyte globulin treatment in patients with aplastic anemia. *N Engl J Med* 1983;308:113–118.
17. Doney K, Pepe M, Storb R et al. Immunosuppressive therapy of aplastic anemia: Results of a prospective, randomized trial of antithymocyte globulin (ATG), methylprednisolone, and oxymethylone to ATG, very high-dose methylprednisolone, and oxymethylone. *Blood* 1992;70:2566–2571.
18. Gluckman E, Esperou-Bourdeau H, Baruchel A et al. Multicenter randomized study comparing cyclosporine A alone and antithymocyte globulin with prednisone for treatment of severe aplastic anemia. *Blood* 1992;79:2540–2546.
19. Lutz P, Gallais C, Albert A et al. Use of intravenous immunoglobulins (IVIg) to treat a child with pancytopenia and hypoplastic marrow. *Ann Hematol* 1992;65:179–200.
20. Geissler K, Forstinger C, Kalhs P et al. Effect of IL-3 on responsiveness to granulocyte-colony stimulating factor in severe aplastic anemia. *Ann Intern Med* 1992;117:223–225.
21. Leoni P, Masia C, Offidani M, Da Lio L. Acycloguanosine for the treatment of aplastic anemia. *Eur J Haematol* 1991;46:120–121.

17

Liver Transplantation for Fulminant Hepatitis B

Ellen B. Hunter and David S. Raiford

CASE PRESENTATION

History of Present Illness

A 28-year-old woman noted the onset of nausea, vomiting, and abdominal pain 10 days before transfer to Vanderbilt University Medical Center. Her physician noted jaundice and she was admitted to hospital. She was taking no medications, vitamins, or food supplements. She reported several needle-stick injuries in her work as a nursing technician in a nursing home, and had received blood transfusions in 1986 at the time of cesarean section. There was no history of I.V. drug or alcohol abuse. Initial laboratory results included total bilirubin 9.6 mg/dL (normal 0.2–1.0), AST 1580 IU/L (normal 10–42), ALT 1720 IU/L (normal 10–60), and serum alkaline phosphatase 108 IU/L (normal 42–121). Hepatitis A IgM antibody and hepatitis C antibodies were not detected. The hepatitis B surface antigen (HBsAg), e antigen (HBeAg), and core antibody (HBcAb) of the IgM class were present in serum. Serologic tests for hepatitis delta were negative. A diagnosis of acute hepatitis B was made and supportive care provided. Progressive deterioration occurred over the ensuing 9 days, with worsening confusion and progressive prolongation of the prothrombin time to 43 s. A CT scan of the head showed no evidence of hemorrhage, edema, or mass. She was transferred to Vanderbilt University Medical Center.

The patient's past medical history included a cesarean section. She smoked one-half pack of cigarettes daily and consumed alcohol infrequently. There was no recognized exposure to known hepatotoxins. Medications on transfer included vitamin K, ranitidine, and lactulose.

Physical Examination

On transfer the patient's blood pressure was 133/62 mm Hg, pulse was 92/min and regular, respiratory rate was 24/min, and rectal temperature was 99.9°F. She was deeply jaundiced but had neither palmar erythema, spider angiomata, nor tattoos. Pupillary constriction to illumination was sluggish but symmetric. The neck was supple and the chest clear to auscultation. Cardiac rhythm was regular and there were no murmurs. The liver was not enlarged to percussion or palpation; shifting dullness and flank bulging were present. Neurologic examination revealed stupor with withdrawal to painful stimuli, intact cranial nerve function, and symmetric reflexes.

Hospital Course

The patient was admitted to the medical intensive care unit with a diagnosis of fulminant hepatic failure due to acute hepatitis B infection. Endotracheal intubation and mechanical ventilation were instituted and a continuous infusion of 10% dextrose was administered by vein. After administration of plasma and cryoprecipitate, a Camino intracranial pressure monitoring catheter was placed in the right frontal area. The initial intracranial pressure (ICP) was 11 mm Hg, with concomitant blood pressure 144/70. The patient's head was kept in the neutral midline position with the head of the bed elevated 30° above horizontal. Mechanical hyperventilation was adjusted to maintain the arterial pCO_2 at 25 mm Hg. Hepatitis B immune globulin (HBIG) was administered I.M. in anticipation of emergent liver transplantation.

The following day an ABO identical donor liver became available. Orthotopic liver transplantation was performed with an operative time of 6 h. Additional HBIG was given during the anhepatic phase of the transplantation surgery. An increase in intracranial pressure to 30 mm Hg during the anhepatic phase responded to I.V. mannitol infusion. The patient received two units of packed red blood cells and six units of fresh frozen plasma during surgery.

On postoperative day 1 the patient was alert and followed commands. The endotracheal tube was removed on postoperative day 2. Steroid responsive allograft rejection developed on postoperative day 6. Vancomycin was administered for 14 days to treat *Staphylococcus au-*

reus bacteremia. Posttransplant, the patient was given HBIG 5 cc I.M. daily for 7 days which resulted in a serum hepatitis B surface antibody level of 6.3 mIU/L, below the target level of 100 mIU/L. The dose of HBIG was increased to 10 cc I.M. daily for 7 days followed by 10 cc I.M. qod for a final week with resultant HBsAb levels ≥100 mIU/L. The serum hepatitis B surface antigen became negative on postoperative day 12. Hepatitis serologies were monitored on a monthly basis. Hepatitis B surface antigen continued to be negative 6 months posttransplant. HBsAb levels remained ≥100 mIU/L without receiving HBIG. At her first anniversary posttransplant evaluation, the patient was clinically stable. However, the HBsAg, HBcAb (Total and IgM), and HBeAg were positive, and the HBsAb and HBeAb were negative. Serum aminotransferase levels were two times the upper limits of normal. A liver biopsy revealed a portal infiltrate without histologic evidence of rejection. These findings were most consistent with recurrent hepatitis B infection and the patient's immunosuppression was decreased. Eighteen months following her transplantation, the patient is clinically stable with mild abnormalities of hepatic biochemical tests. She has persistent hepatitis B infection.

FULMINANT HEPATIC FAILURE

Definition and Background

Fulminant hepatic failure (FHF) is among the most dramatic and challenging entities encountered in clinical medicine. As defined by Trey and Davidson [1], FHF is a syndrome of severe acute hepatic dysfunction occurring in patients with no history of antecedent liver disease in which hepatic encephalopathy develops within 8 weeks of the onset of the illness. Currently, this definition has been narrowed further in that many experienced clinicians feel that significant impairment of coagulation function must be present to establish this diagnosis. Approximately 2000 cases of FHF occur annually in the United States and the historical mortality of this condition is 70–80%. The formidable nature of this syndrome is largely attributable to its abruptness, unpredictability, and potential for a myriad of serious complications. That spontaneous recovery with complete restoration of hepatic function occurs in a significant minority of patients underscores the deliberative and management challenges for physicians treating these patients.

Whereas in the United States the leading cause of FHF is viral hepatitis, acetaminophen-induced hepatic necrosis accounts for the majority of cases in the United Kingdom [2, 3]. The balance of cases of FHF are generally due to drug toxicity, toxin-related injuries, or rare metabolic disorders. When possible, defining the etiology of FHF is of great importance for several reasons. First, specific antidotal therapy (e.g., *N*-acetylcysteine for acetaminophen toxicity) may alter the natural history of the syndrome. Second, there are important public health issues to be pursued when acute viral hepatitis is diagnosed. Third, the prognosis in FHF is linked to the etiology of the syndrome [3]. Historically, patients with FHF due to acetaminophen hepatotoxicity and hepatitis A have had a more favorable prognosis (50–60% survival) than patients with hepatitis B (20–40% survival). The bleakest prognosis has been that for patients with FHF due to non-A, non-B hepatitis or idiosyncratic drug hepatotoxicity (10–15% survival) [4].

Complications and Management of Fulminant Hepatic Failure

The complications of FHF may occur precipitously, are multisystem in nature, are unpredictable but occur in limited combinations, and can be life-threatening. The importance of prompt recognition of this syndrome and initiation of skilled supportive care by those experienced in the management of this condition cannot be overemphasized. Optimally, once the diagnosis of FHF is suspected or established, strong consideration should be given to urgent transfer of the patient to a medical center where liver transplantation is available if needed. The most frequent complications of FHF include cerebral edema, coagulopathy, hemodynamic instability, renal insufficiency, hypoglycemia, infection, and acid-base/electrolyte disorders. Supportive management of FHF should be rendered in an intensive care unit. Discussion of the details of this supportive management are beyond the scope of this chapter, but several excellent reviews are available [5–7]. Special emphasis should be placed on identifying, if possible, the etiology of FHF. The history must be meticulous in searching for risks for viral hepatitis, for exposure to recognized hepatotoxins (e.g., acetaminophen, drugs, halogenated hydrocarbons, and wild mushrooms such as *Amanita phalloides*). Physical findings will include delirium, jaundice, ecchymosis, and a diminished area of hepatic percussion dullness, in any combination. Examination of serum for antibody (IgM) to hepatitis A, hepatitis B surface antigen and (IgM) core antibody, antibody to HIV, ceruloplasmin level (if the patient is under 50 years old), and acetaminophen level is mandatory. As seroconversion occurs relatively late in the course of primary hepatitis C infection, antibody tests are less reliable in diagnosis. Detection of hepatitis C RNA in serum using the polymerase chain reaction may permit specific diagnosis of acute hepatitic C viral (HCV) infection.

Initial management includes admission to the intensive care unit, provision of I.V. dextrose and H_2 blockers, and serial assessment of the patient's mental status, vital signs, and urine output. Specific antidotal treatment is initiated for acetaminophen or mushroom poisoning. Deliberations concerning the suitability of liver transplantation as a potential therapy for the patient should begin soon after admission because the time course of deterioration that might prompt the need for transplantation may be rapid. The prothrombin time, monitored serially, is of great prognostic value, and unless clinical bleeding is present, the prophylactic use of plasma products is discouraged. Clinical evidence of cerebral edema, hemodynamic instability, oliguria, or infection should prompt rapid and aggressive treatment. The particular importance of maintaining adequate cerebral perfusion may warrant direct measurement of intracranial pressure in patients felt likely to come to transplantation [2]. It is well to remember that with excellent supportive care, spontaneous and complete recovery from this dread condition is possible.

Prognostic Assessment/Role of Liver Transplantation

The management of FHF has been altered significantly since the advent of liver transplantation. Historically, the majority of patients who developed FHF died despite heroic supportive intensive care. Today, the majority of patients with FHF who are treated with liver transplantation survive. Although, intuitively liver transplantation is the most definitive therapy to remedy the consequences of sudden loss of functional hepatic mass, its benefits are unlikely ever to be established as the result of a controlled clinical trial [7, 8]. Practical dilemmas for clinicians include determining whether and when to proceed to liver replacement with its attendant lifelong consequences for a condition in which spontaneous and complete recovery is possible. These complex deliberations occur within a period of hours to days and are dynamic in that they are influenced greatly by the patient's clinical course. Optimally, consideration of the issues surrounding transplantation should begin immediately upon recognition that an individual patient has FHF. For practical reasons, identifying any existing contraindications to liver transplantation should assume priority early. In addition to the usual contraindications applied when considering elective liver transplantation, patients with FHF must be assessed serially for evidence of irreversible brain injury, infection, and deterioration in cardiopulmonary function which would preclude successful operative management.

Assessment of prognosis has been facilitated by guidelines developed through retrospective multivariate analysis in a large series of patients with FHF seeking clinical correlates with fatality. These guidelines have subsequently been validated prospectively [3]. Although a general consensus has not been reached, most clinicians would agree that if the estimated likelihood of survival for an individual patient is less than 15–20%, then liver transplantation is indicated [6, 9]. Risk stratification in FHF allows selection of patients who are least likely to recover spontaneously. Present prognostic guidelines divide patients with FHF into two groups: those with acetaminophen toxicity and those with FHF due to other causes. As developed by O'Grady et al. [3], death is likely (>80% probability) for patients with acetaminophen toxicity in two instances: (i) those who have an arterial blood pH < 7.30 or (ii) those who have a prothrombin time >100 s, serum creatinine > 3.4 mg/dl, and grade III or IV encephalopathy. For patients with FHF due to causes other than acetaminophen, the likelihood of death without transplantation is >90% when any three of the following five criteria are present:

   (i)   age <10 or >40 years
  (ii)   duration of jaundice >1 week before development of encephalopathy
 (iii)   serum bilirubin concentration >18 mg/dl
 (iv)   etiology of FHF is non-A, non-B hepatitis or drug/toxin
  (v)   prothrombin time >50 s.

Approximately two-thirds of patients listed for liver transplantation in the setting of FHF will come to transplantation with a mean waiting time of approximately 3 days. The balance of patients activated for transplantation will die before a donor organ is available, will develop a contraindication precluding transplantation, or rarely will recover spontaneously. Specific considerations in the peritransplant management of individual patients depends on the etiology of the FHF, on the clinical course, and on patient factors. The successful application of liver transplantation for FHF has improved the prognosis for selected patients who are unlikely to survive without transplantation. Transplantation series spanning the period from 1985 to 1990 report mean survival likelihoods at 1 year in the range 65–70% [6, 9]. More recent data suggest that rates approaching 80% may be achievable today [6, 7].

LIVER TRANSPLANTATION FOR HEPATITIS B

Background

Hepatitis B is a worldwide health problem affecting 300 million persons. Despite the availability of an effective vaccine, it is estimated that

300,000 new cases occur each year in the United States [10]. Of adult patients with acute hepatitis B infection, fewer than 1% will develop FHF. The mortality of patients with fulminant hepatitis B in one series was 61% [11]. In addition to the serious complications of FHF, 5% of adult patients with acute hepatitis B will progress to chronic hepatitis. The risk of chronicity is significantly higher in the neonate, where the frequency approaches 90%. The complications of chronic hepatitis B include cirrhosis—with associated variceal bleeding, ascites, and encephalopathy—and hepatocellular carcinoma. It has been estimated that 4000–6000 chronic hepatitis B patients in the United States die each year from cirrhosis or primary hepatocellular carcinoma. Patients with liver failure from fulminant hepatitis B or end-stage chronic hepatitis B represent a significant number of patients who are potential candidates for orthotopic liver transplantation. However, concerns regarding recurrent infection in the allograft have limited the widespread use of this treatment option.

Clinical Characteristics of Recurrent Hepatitis B Infection

The risk of hepatitis B virus (HBV) recurrence following transplantation is significant. Fifty-nine patients with HBV infection were transplanted at the University of Pittsburgh for fulminant hepatitis B ($n = 8$) and postnecrotic cirrhosis ($n = 51$) [12]. Eighty-two percent of patients who survived at least 60 days had recurrent hepatitis B infection. A negative pretransplant hepatitis B e antigen (HBeAg), suggesting lower viral replication, was associated with a decreased risk for hepatitis B recurrence. The clinical course of posttransplant patients with recurrent hepatitis B ranges from fulminant hepatic failure to chronic hepatitis with subsequent development of cirrhosis. In transplant patients with recurrent hepatitis B, the progression to cirrhosis appears accelerated in comparison to nonimmunosuppressed hepatitis B patients. This may be due, in part, to enhanced viral replication in the setting of immunosuppression. Virus causing allograft reinfection is believed to come from extrahepatic reservoirs of infection. Investigators have detected hepatitis B virus in peripheral mononuclear cells, spleen, kidneys, and pancreas [13, 14]. A unique histologic entity, termed fibrosing cholestatic hepatitis (FCH), has been reported in a small subset of patients with recurrent hepatitis B [15]. The histologic features include periportal fibrosis, cholestasis, and ballooning of hepatocytes with minimal inflammation. FCH is associated with a dismal prognosis in that patients develop rapidly progressive liver failure. A patient retransplanted with liver failure due to recurrent hepatitis B and FCH had recurrent FCH 4 weeks posttransplant and died [16].

Prevention and Treatment of Recurrent Hepatitis B

Strategies to prevent HBV infection of the transplanted liver have included hepatitis B immunoglobulins (HBIG), antiviral therapy, and xenograft transplantation. HBIG has been administered in an attempt to neutralize circulating HBV particles. Short-term administration in the perioperative period delays but does not prevent recurrence of hepatitis B infection [17]. In an uncontrolled trial reported by Samuel et al., 110 HBsAg positive patients received liver transplantation [18]. Patients received 10,000 IU of HBIG intravenously during the anhepatic phase and daily for 6 days postoperatively. Subsequently, patients received additional doses of HBIG intravenously to maintain antibody levels to hepatitis B surface antigen above 100 mIU/L during follow-up. All patients became HBsAg negative during the first postoperative week. However, during the mean follow-up of 19.6 months, 25 (22.7%) of patients became positive for HBsAg. Recurrence of HBsAg was influenced by the pretransplant liver disease. The 2-year actuarial recurrence rate of HBsAg after transplantation was 59% for posthepatitis B cirrhosis, 13% for posthepatitis B-delta cirrhosis, and 0% for fulminant hepatitis B. HBV DNA positive patients had a 96% risk of recurrence at 2 years versus 29% in the HBV DNA negative patients. In a large, retrospective study from 17 European centers, 334 HBsAg positive patients who underwent liver transplantation were followed for evidence of recurrence [19]. Patients received long-term immunoprophylaxis ($\geq$6 months), short-term immunoprophylaxis ($\leq$2 months), or no treatment with HBIG. The 3-year actuarial risk of recurrence for all patients was 50%. Patients transplanted for HBV-related cirrhosis had the highest risk of recurrence of 67% versus 17% for patients with fulminant HBV infection. The presence of HBV DNA in the serum at the time of transplant increased the risk of recurrence. Independent predictors of a low risk of HBV recurrence were the long-term administration of HBIG, hepatitis delta virus superinfection, and acute liver disease. Based on these studies, long-term HBIG administration may be beneficial in preventing HBV recurrence and prolonging survival posttransplant. The cost of long-term parenteral HBIG is estimated at $15,000 for the first year.

In an effort to inhibit viral replication, antiviral therapy has been used both pretransplant and posttransplant. Interferon-α-2b is approved for chronic hepatitis B at a dose of 5 million units subcutaneously given daily for 4 months. It has been shown to inhibit viral replication in approximately 40% of patients [20]. Its use is relatively contraindicated in cirrhotic patients because of myelosuppressive effects and the induction of immune-mediated hepatocyte injury which could lead to hepatic decompensation. It has been postulated that using lower doses of interferon-alfa reduces viral activity and decreases the risk of posttransplant recurrence. Two patients with hepatitis B-related cirrhosis at the Mayo Clinic were treated during the pretransplantation period with interferon-alfa-2a, 1.5 million units daily. Postoperatively the dose was increased to 3 million units daily for 3 months [21]. Pretransplant, the patients were HBV DNA positive in the serum by a molecular hybridization assay. Serum HBsAg remained positive posttransplant, and HBV DNA levels in the serum increased. The patients subsequently developed chronic hepatitis, and one patient required retransplantation for allograft failure due to HBV infection. A recent study evaluated the effect of pretransplant treatment with interferon-α-2b, 3 million units thrice weekly in 22 patients with hepatitis B-related cirrhosis awaiting transplantation in comparison to 26 untreated historical patients with hepatitis B-related cirrhosis who underwent transplantation [22]. Posttransplant, patients in both groups received long-term HBIG. Eight of the 22 patients treated with interferon required a dose reduction because of severe myelosuppression (e.g., neutropenia less than $800/mm^3$ and thrombocytopenia less than $50,000/mm^3$). Seven of the eight HBV-DNA positive patients treated with interferon became negative. Two of these patients clinically improved during interferon therapy and did not require transplantation. However, the rate of HBV reinfection posttransplantation was not significantly different between the interferon-treated and untreated groups (44% vs. 58%). Treatment with interferon did not delay the onset of HBV reinfection. Because of interferon's immunostimulating effects, concerns about the potential for precipitating allograft rejection has limited its use in the posttransplant period. In a preliminary report, 13 patients received interferon-alfa 2b, 3 million units three times weekly for recurrent hepatitis B posttransplant [23]. Seroconversion or improvement in aminotransferase levels did not occur in this group of patients. Interferon administration was not associated with increased frequency of allograft rejection. Other antiviral agents presently being evaluated in allograft recipients with recurrent hepatitis B include adenine arabinoside monophosphate (Ara-AMP) [24]. In a pilot study, eight patients received Ara-AMP at a dose of 10 mg/kg/day for 5 days followed by 5 mg/kg/day for 23 days by intramuscular injection twice daily. Antiviral effects were observed with decreased viral replication. However, the effects were transient and HBV DNA reappeared once the drug was discontinued. Reversible myalgias occurred in two patients and required temporary discontinuation of the drug.

In an attempt to prevent hepatitis B virus recurrence, xenotransplantation has been considered. Baboon livers appear to be resistant to HBV infection. In 1992, Starzl et al. performed the first baboon-to-human liver xenotransplantation in a 35-year-old man coinfected with HBV and HIV [25]. Postoperatively the patient's course was complicated by multiple infections, renal failure, and cholestasis. The patient died 70 days posttransplant of intracranial hemorrhage due to angioinvasive aspergillus infection. There was no evidence of recurrent HBV infection in the short follow-up period by immunohistochemical staining for hepatitis B surface or core antigen in the xenograft. Further studies are needed to elucidate the recurrence rate of HBV in xenografts.

SUMMARY

Herein, we present the case of a 28-year-old woman with fulminant hepatitis B who was treated with liver transplantation. She received short-term HBIG but had hepatitis B recurrence 11 months following transplantation. Recurrence of hepatitis B occurs frequently posttransplant and patients may develop significant liver dysfunction over a short period of time. Risk for recurrence appears lowest in patients with fulminant hepatitis B and in those with chronic hepatitis B infection without active viral replication (manifest by the absence of HBV DNA and HBeAg in serum) at the time of transplantation. Administration of HBIG to maintain HBsAb levels ≥ 100 mIU/L lessens the likelihood of allograft dysfunction due to infection by HBV and appears to increase survival likelihood at 5 years posttransplant. Enthusiasm for this therapy has been tempered by its expense and need for chronic administration. At present, many liver transplant programs consider the presence of HBV DNA or HBeAg in serum to be strong contraindications to hepatic replacement for chronic liver disease. Based on presently available data, it appears reasonable to limit liver transplantation for hepatitis B to patients with acute infection who develop fulminant hepatic failure or those with chronic infection who are HBV DNA and HBeAg negative. Long-term parenteral administration of HBIG to maintain HBsAb levels ≥ 100 mIU/L is the best available prophylaxis against reinfection posttransplant and should be given. Antiviral therapies such as interferon and nucleoside analogues are presently being evaluated in the hope that they might enhance the long-term prognosis for patients treated with liver transplantation for hepatitis B-related liver disease.

REFERENCES

1. Trey C, Davidson CS. The management of fulminant hepatic failure. In: Popper H, Schaffner F, eds. *Progress in Liver Diseases*. Vol. III. New York: Grune & Stratton, 1970:282–298.

2. Lidofsky SD, Bass NM, Prager MC, et al. Intracranial pressure monitoring and liver transplantation for fulminant hepatic failure. *Hepatology* 1992;16:1–7.

3. O'Grady JG, Alexander GJM, Hayllar KM et al. Early indicators of prognosis in fulminant hepatic failure. *Gastroenterology* 1989;97:439–445.

4. Hughes RD, Wendon J, Gimson AES. Acute liver failure. *Gut* 1991(Suppl.)^{8}6–S91.

5. Fingerote RJ, Bain VG. Fulminant hepatic failure. *Am J Gastroenterol* 1993;88:1000–1010.

6. Lee WM. Acute liver failure. *N Engl J Med* 1993;329:1862–1872.

7. Muñoz SJ. Difficult management problems in fulminant hepatic failure. *Semin Liver Dis* 1993;13:395–413.

8. Berman J, O'Grady J, Elias E et al. Transplantation for fulminant hepatic failure. *Lancet* 1990;335:407–409.

9. Lidofsky SD. Liver transplantation for fulminant hepatic failure. *Gastroenterol Clin N Amer* 1993;22:257–269.

10. CDC. Protection against viral hepatitis. Recommendations of the Immunizing Practices Advisory Committee (ACIP). *MMWR* 1990;39:1–26.

11. O'Grady JG, Gimson AES, O'Brien CJ. Controlled trials of charcoal hemoperfusion and prognostic factors in fulminant hepatic failure. *Gastroenterology* 1988;94:1186–1192.

12. Todo S, Demetris AJ, Van Thiel D, et al. Orthotopic liver transplantation for patients with hepatitis B virus-related liver disease. *Hepatology* 1991;13:619–626.

13. Féray C, Zignego AL, Samuel D et al. Persistent hepatitis B virus infection of mononuclear blood cells without concomitant liver infection. *Transplantation* 1990;49:1155–1158.

14. Yotte B, Burns DK, Bhatta HS et al. Extrahepatic hepatitis B virus DNA sequence in patients with acute hepatitis B infection. *Hepatology* 1990;12:187–192.

15. Davies SE, Portmann BC, O'Grady JG et al. Hepatic histologic findings after transplantation for chronic hepatitis B virus infection, including a unique pattern of fibrosing cholestatic hepatitis. *Hepatology* 1991;13:150–157.

16. Benner KG, Lee RG, Keefe EB et al. Fibrosing cytolytic liver failure secondary to recurrent hepatitis B after liver transplantation. *Gastroenterology* 1992;103:1307–1312.

17. O'Grady JG, Smith HM, Davies SE. Hepatitis B virus reinfection after orthotopic liver transplantation: Serological and clinical implications. *J Hepatol* 1992;14:104–111.

18. Samuel D, Bismuth A, Mathieu D et al. Passive immunoprophylaxis after liver transplantation in HBsAg-positive patients. *Lancet* 1991; 337:813–815.

19. Samuel D, Muller R, Alexander G et al. Liver transplantation in European patients with hepatitis B surface antigen. *N Engl J Med* 1993;329:1842–1847.

20. Perrillo RB, Schiff ER, Davis GL et al. A randomized, controlled trial of Interferon Alfa-2b alone and after Prednisone withdrawal for the treatment of chronic hepatitis B. *N Engl J Med* 1990;323:295–301.

21. Douglas DP, Rakela J, Taswell HF et al. Hepatitis B virus replication patterns after orthotopic liver transplantation: De novo versus recurrent infection. *Transplant Proc* 1993;25:1755–1757.

22. Marcellin P, Samuel D, Areias J et al. Pretransplantation interferon treatment and recurrence of hepatitis B virus infection after liver transplantation for hepatitis B-related end-stage liver disease. *Hepatology* 1994;19:6–12.

23. Wright HI, Gavalar JS, Van Thiel DH. Preliminary experience with α-2b-interferon therapy of viral hepatitis in liver allograft recipients. *Transplantation* 1992;53:121–123.

24. Marcellin P, Samuel D, Loriot A et al. Antiviral effects of adenine arabinoside monophosphate (Ara-AMP) in patients with recurrence of hepatitis B virus (HBV) infection after liver transplantation. *Hepatology* 1990;12:966A.

25. Starzl TE, Fung J, Tzakis A et al. Baboon-to-human liver transplantation. *Lancet* 1993;341:65–71.

18

Variceal Hemorrhage Following Liver Transplantation

Richard R. Lopez, David S. Raiford,
and C. Wright Pinson

CASE PRESENTATION

History of the Present Illness

A 38-year-old woman with primary biliary cirrhosis, progressive hepatic dysfunction, and portal hypertension was admitted to the hospital with recurrent variceal hemorrhage. For 2 years she suffered multiple episodes of gastrointestinal bleeding from esophageal varices. Despite sclerotherapy she continued to bleed intermittently. Because of recurrent variceal bleeding, she underwent a distal splenorenal shunt (DSRS) and coronary vein ligation. This successfully decompressed the esophageal varices; however, 10 months later she developed recurrent bleeding from gastric varices. Her liver function remained stable with mild to moderate excretory dysfunction but normal synthetic function. A splenic artery arteriogram demonstrated patency of the DSRS, but esophagogastroduodenoscopy (EGD) revealed large, bleeding gastric varices.

Because of life-threatening hemorrhage from the gastric varices, a transjugular intrahepatic portasystemic shunt (TIPS) was placed utilizing an 8-mm Wall stent. After TIPS placement, portal vein pressures decreased from 35 to 23 mm Hg, and there was a decrease in the gradient between portal and hepatic vein pressures from 27 to 5 mm Hg and she stopped bleeding. Because of her precarious clinical condition, she was placed on the waiting list for liver transplantation.

One month later she developed new epigastric and left upper quadrant discomfort, progressive ascites, and peripheral edema. A Doppler ultrasound revealed thrombus within the TIPS and the extrahepatic portal vein. Magnetic resonance angiography confirmed portal vein thrombosis and showed patency of the superior mesenteric vein (SMV) and the DSRS. Repeat EGD revealed large gastric varices. One week later, she underwent orthotopic liver transplantation (OLTX). At the time of her operation she was found to have extreme adhesions in the left upper quadrant as a result of her previous shunt operation. Her native portal vein was small and thrombosed while the SMV was thick walled but patent. Because of the portal vein thrombosis, an interposition vein graft (donor iliac vein) was placed between the donor portal vein and the recipient SMV. This vein graft was placed retropancreatic in the normal position of the portal vein and anastomosed end to end to the recipient SMV. The donor common hepatic artery was anastomosed end to end to the recipient common hepatic artery, and biliary reconstruction was with an end to end choledochocholedochostomy.

The patient's initial postoperative course was uneventful. The hepatic allograft functioned immediately and she was extubated on postoperative day (POD) 2. A Doppler ultrasound on POD 1 revealed a patent portal vein and hepatic artery. On POD 2, there was no evidence of intraabdominal or gastrointestinal bleeding and, therefore, a heparin infusion was initiated at a dose of 10 IU/kg/h. On that day, her prothrombin time (PT) was 14 s and platelet count was 43,000. By POD 11 her total bilirubin had decreased to 2.1 mg/dl, her aspartate aminotransferase (AST) was normal at 31 IU/L, and her alanine aminotransferase (ALT) was twice normal at 89 IU/L. She was ambulating, tolerating a regular diet, and preparing for discharge. She was started on warfarin and plans were made for long-term anticoagulation.

The following day her serum aminotransferase levels increased significantly and she complained of mild abdominal discomfort and increased abdominal girth.

Physical Examination

The patient's vital signs were as follows:

Temperature	99.4°F
Pulse	100/min
Blood pressure	140/80 mm Hg

Respiratory rate   16/min
Weight   46.8 kg

The patient was alert and oriented. Her sclerae were slightly icteric and the remainder of the head and neck examination was unremarkable. Her lungs were clear to auscultation and percussion and her heart rate was regular with normal heart tones. The abdomen was moderately distended with fluid and slightly tender to palpation over the hepatic allograft. The incision was intact without signs of infection or dehiscence. A standard biliary T-tube exited below the incision. She had moderate edema in her lower extremities but no calf tenderness. Neurological examination was unremarkable.

Laboratory Evaluation

The laboratory findings were as follows:

	POD 11	POD 12
Hematocrit (%)	25	36
WBC (/hpf)	14,000	8,200
Platelet count (/hpf)	98,000	51,000
BUN (mg/dl)	33	23
Creatinine (mg/dl)	0.6	0.7
Glucose (g/dl)	222	336
Total bilirubin (g/dl)	2.1	2.8
Alkaline phosphatase (IU/L)	121	123
LDH (IU/L)	233	4030
AST (IU/L)	31	2130
ALT (IU/L)	89	1810
CSA level (ng/ml)	114	210

Hospital Course

A transfascial allograft liver biopsy showed centrilobular necrosis consistent with ischemia (Fig. 18-1). A flow signal could not be demonstrated within the portal vein by Doppler ultrasound, although flow signals were identified from within the hepatic artery, hepatic veins, and vena cava. Moderate ascites was noted. She subsequently developed hematemesis, and EGD revealed gastric varices with evidence of recent bleeding but no esophageal varices. Angiography with delayed venous

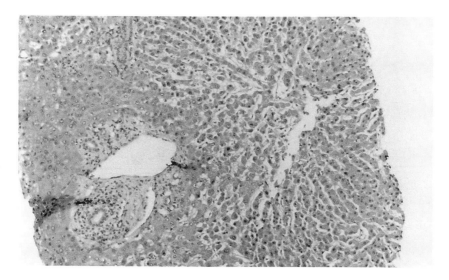

Figure 18-1.   Liver biopsy shows centrilobular necrosis.

phase confirmed the presence of a portal vein thrombosis, a patent DSRS, and a patent SMV. She was returned to the operating room where she was found to have acute thrombosis of the donor portal vein and the interposition vein graft with propagation into the SMV. The hepatic artery was patent. A portal vein thrombectomy was carried out, and flow through the portal vein was reestablished. Because of concern about rethrombosis, a large gastroduodenal varix was diverted and anastomosed end to side to the donor portal vein as well.

She tolerated the operation well, and over the next week her liver function improved and she had no further evidence of gastrointestinal bleeding. Heparin was reinstituted 24 h after the operation, and later, long-term anticoagulation continued with warfarin. A follow-up Doppler ultrasound of the allograft and porta hepatitis revealed hepatopetal flow in the portal vein. The patient was anticoagulated for 1 year and is doing well 2 years after the transplant. She has had no allograft dysfunction or variceal bleeding.

DISCUSSION OF THE DIFFERENTIAL DIAGNOSIS

The case presented is that of a woman with severe portal hypertension and progressive liver failure due to primary biliary cirrhosis. She underwent urgent OLTX after a TIPS failed in achieving sustained decompression of the portal venous system and she developed recurrent life-threatening variceal hemorrhage. Prior to attempts at decompressing the splanchnic venous system, this patient was felt to be an excellent transplant candidate, as she was young and without other significant medical problems. The most significant manifestation of her liver disease was portal hypertension. In the majority of transplant candidates with portal hypertension, variceal hemorrhage can be controlled with sclerotherapy. However, some patients will need portal decompression. In this patient, attempts to alleviate life-threatening variceal hemorrhage included selective and intrahepatic portasystemic shunts. A DSRS is usually effective at decompressing esophageal varices, but patients may subsequently develop gastric varices. Two advantages of the DSRS in a transplant candidate are the lower incidence of hepatic encephalopathy postshunt and no increase in surgical risk of transplantation because dissection in the porta hepatitis is avoided. Transjugular intrahepatic portasystemic shunt placement is generally successful in lowering portal pressures enough to stop variceal hemorrhage. As with any invasive procedure, there are associated risks including bleeding during placement of the shunt and thrombosis. If thrombosis occurs, the patient is at high risk for rebleeding from varices, and the thrombus may propagate into the extrahepatic portal vein, which can complicate a transplant operation.

Thus, this patient's transplant operation was complicated by both pretransplant and posttransplant portal vein thrombosis. This necessitated thrombectomy and placement of a venous conduit from the recipient SMV to the donor portal vein. Because of the preexistent thrombus in the extrahepatic portal vein and SMV, the patient was at increased risk for rethrombosis posttransplant.

It is helpful to differentiate posttransplant complications based on when they occur: early versus late. Early complications generally refers to those occurring within 30 days of transplant. The major categories of early complications are listed in Table 18-1.

Table 18-1. Early Posttransplant Complications

Hemorrhage	Intraabdominal, gastrointestinal, wound
Vascular	Stenosis, thrombosis
Biliary	Leak, obstruction
Intestinal	Perforation, obstruction
Wound	Dehiscence, hematoma, lymphocele
Infection	Bacterial, fungal, viral
Rejection	Acute

Although the patient's initial postoperative course was uneventful, she developed abruptly elevations in hepatic biochemical tests, a change in her physical examination, and recurrent variceal hemorrhage. Examination of the changes in her biochemical profile revealed a significant rise in serum aminotransferase levels and lactate dehydrogenase but only a slight increase in serum bilirubin and no increase in alkaline phosphatase. This biochemical pattern indicates severe hepatocellular injury with minimal effect on biliary epithelium. Such a pattern of injury can be seen with ischemia or severe rejection, although with rejection there is usually a more significant rise in the serum bilirubin. In addition, patients with acute rejection often have a leukocytosis and may suffer systemic manifestation such as fever, myalgias, arthralgias, and headache. The precipitous, marked elevations in serum aminotransferase levels observed were most consistent with ischemia. In the newly transplanted liver, ischemia may be due to hepatic artery thrombosis, portal vein thrombosis, or rarely to hepatic venous outflow obstruction.

Other important diagnoses in the differential include biliary tract complications and infection, particularly intraabdominal infection. Serum aminotransferase and bilirubin levels may increase in response to intraabdominal infection, but usually the rise is mild to moderate and the patient often experiences other systemic manifestations such as fever, hemodynamic changes, or leukocytosis. Biliary tract complications may also affect serum aminotransferase levels but usually have the greatest effect on serum bilirubin and alkaline phosphatase. As expected, these biochemical changes are most marked in patients with biliary obstruction. Clinical symptoms associated with biliary tract complications vary from localized abdominal tenderness to cholangitis and sepsis. Because of immunosuppression, clinical signs and symptoms are often delayed and blunted. Abdominal tenderness can be seen with any postoperative complication and must be evaluated in conjunction with other clinical changes and blood chemistries.

Posttransplant gastrointestinal hemorrhage may be due to varices, ulceration, angiodysplasia, colitis, or surgical trauma (i.e., anastomotic sites). Posttransplant hemorrhage from esophageal varices in a patient with a DSRS should raise concern about the possibility of shunt dysfunction or thrombosis, especially if accompanied by sudden decreases in white blood cell count and platelet count. In this particular patient, the history of pretransplant portal vein thrombosis, posttransplant hemorrhage from gastric rather than esophageal varices, development of ascites, and severe allograft dysfunction led to suspicion of portal vein thrombosis.

In the setting of early posttransplant variceal hemorrhage and allograft dysfunction, several diagnostic maneuvers must be accomplished urgently. Because rejection is common after OLTX, a transfascial liver biopsy was the first diagnostic procedure performed and revealed centrilobular necrosis (Fig. 18-1), which is the classic injury pattern for ischemia. This pattern of injury reflects the increased susceptibility of hepatocytes around the central vein to hypoperfusion and hypoxia. In general, periportal parenchyma is preserved except in the most severe cases of ischemic injury. Acute cellular rejection has a distinctly different histological pattern. Typically, there is expansion of the portal tracts with mononuclear cells, lymphocytes, and, frequently, eosinophils. In addition, there is invasion and damage of the bile duct epithelium and vascular endothelium by lymphocytes.

Doppler ultrasonography is very helpful in assessing vascular patency posttransplant with an accuracy of greater than 90% [1]. In this patient, it did not detect flow in the portal vein but demonstrated pulsatile flow in the hepatic artery, patent hepatic veins, and vena cava, and confirmed the presence of ascites. Angiography will confirm the presence of arterial or venous thrombosis; however, in the acute setting, the transplant surgeon may elect to proceed with surgical exploration based on the results of the Doppler ultrasound and the extent of allograft dysfunction. Further diagnostic tests should be based on the level of suspicion for a specific complication. If there had been concern about a biliary complication or intraabdominal infection, cholangiography and computed tomography of the abdomen could have been performed. For patients with gastrointestinal hemorrhage, endoscopy may be helpful in delineating the source of bleeding and, in selected patients, therapeutic maneuvers attempted. The presence of varices indicates splanchnic venous hypertension.

The clinical presentation of early hepatic artery thrombosis is variable. It can appear similar to biliary obstruction or to fulminant hepatic failure. In severe cases, the patient develops fever, hemodynamic instability, respiratory distress and sepsis from enteric organisms due to acute hepatic failure. Survival in these patients depends on urgent retransplantation. In other patients, hepatic necrosis may be limited and the allograft will survive. However, as the biliary tract is dependent on arterial flow, these patients almost invariably develop biliary tract complications. The spectrum of biliary tract complications associated with hepatic artery thrombosis ranges from failure to heal the anastomosis to multiple biliary strictures. Frequently, these complications lead to infection such as cholangitis or intraabdominal abscess.

As with hepatic artery thrombosis, the clinical presentation of early portal vein thrombosis is variable and includes fulminant hepatic failure, allograft dysfunction, progressive ascites, and variceal bleeding (in the setting of preexisting varices). Even in patients in whom allograft dysfunction is mild to moderate, variceal hemorrhage may be life-threatening. In patients without predisposing factors, one should investigate the possibility of a hypercoagulable state. Therapy is directed at reestablishing portal inflow to the transplanted liver which necessitates prompt surgical intervention. Late portal vein thrombosis has much less effect on allograft function, provided there is adequate arterial inflow. The principal sequela of this late complication is variceal hemorrhage.

DIAGNOSIS

The diagnosis was posttransplant portal vein thrombosis.

DISCUSSION

This case illustrates several important issues that challenge the clinician and warrant further discussion. These include

1.   Management of portal hypertension in transplant candidates
2.   Operative management of portal vein thrombosis
3.   Posttransplant management of portal vein thrombosis

Over the past 10 years, management of portal hypertension has changed principally as a result of liver transplantation. Liver transplantation is indicated as treatment for end-stage liver disease but not usually for portal hypertension alone. Portal hypertension has various etiologies, including a number of diseases in which hepatic function is preserved. Thus, management decisions depend on assessments of the etiology and severity of liver disease and of candidacy for liver replacement. Our patient was an excellent transplant candidate and, therefore, her portal hypertension was managed with the expectation that she would eventually undergo liver replacement. Therapeutic options included the use of β-blockers, vasodilators, vasopressin, octreotide, balloon tamponade, endoscopic sclerotherapy, and a portasystemic shunt. The majority of patients with bleeding from esophageal varices can be successfully managed acutely with sclerotherapy. Bleeding from gastric varices presents a more formidable problem due to the relative lack of efficacy and higher risk for complication of endoscopic sclerotherapy. The real challenge occurs in the patient who fails sclerotherapy and needs portal decompression. For transplant candidates, the goal of therapy is temporizing the patient's condition until transplantation. This is unlike the nontransplant candidate for whom the goal of therapy is to reduce permanently the portal hypertension to prevent further variceal bleeding.

In transplant candidates, portal decompression can be achieved with a surgical shunt, either selective or central, a TIPS, or liver transplantation. If one elects to proceed with a nontransplant procedure, the procedure should effectively reduce portal pressures without impacting significantly on the future transplant operation. Such treatment can be achieved with a DSRS or a mesocaval shunt in which dissection within the porta hepatis is avoided. Unlike the DSRS, the central shunt needs to be ligated at the time of transplantation to ensure adequate mesenteric venous inflow to the hepatic allograft. Several transplant centers have reported similar results following transplantation in patients with and without portasystemic shunts [2, 3].

Alternatively, patients may undergo a TIPS. This small-caliber intrahepatic shunt is usually successful in lowering portal venous pressure enough to stop variceal bleeding; however, complications may arise. Ring et al. [4] reported successful placement of TIPS in 13 transplant candidates, 7 of whom had OLTX within 4 months. Four patients stabilized after the TIPS and were followed expectantly. Only one patient rebled $3\frac{1}{2}$ months after shunt placement as a result of shunt occlusion caused by neointimal proliferation. At Vanderbilt Medical Center, 56% of patients who had a TIPS developed shunt stenosis or occlusion within 6 months. Furthermore, 67% of the patients with stenosis or occlusion rebled from varices [5]. Thus, we have used TIPS as a bridge to transplantation, realizing that long-term patency is limited. This patient represents the most severe complication of TIPS. Not only did she rebleed after shunt thrombosis but thrombus propagated into the extrahepatic portal vein and SMV, which significantly complicated the transplant operation. In addition, it predisposed her to rethrombosis posttransplant.

Urgent liver transplantation is an option for patients with refractory variceal bleeding and advanced cirrhosis. The Pittsburgh group has reported excellent results with OLTX for patients with variceal hemorrhage [6]. The real issue in patients who are acutely bleeding is whether the bleeding can be controlled long enough to obtain a suitable donor liver.

Another aspect highlighted by this case is the operative management of portal vein thrombosis; during the transplant operation and posttransplant. Initially, the transplanted liver is dependent on inflow from the hepatic artery and the portal vein. Because of this requirement, portal vein thrombosis was initially felt to be a contraindication to liver transplantation. However, with improved surgical techniques, patients with isolated portal vein thrombosis can undergo successful liver transplantation. The surgical techniques that have been described include portal vein thrombectomy, retrograde dissection of the portal vein to the confluence of the SMV and splenic vein, and the use of donor vein, usually the iliac vein, as an interposition graft from the SMV to the portal vein. Additionally, if the transplant surgeon anticipates a prolonged difficult portal vein reconstruction, the hepatic artery can be reconstructed first. Perhaps the greatest challenge to the transplant surgeon is the patient with extensive thrombosis of the splanchnic venous system. In most instances this would be considered a contraindication to liver transplantation; however, there are anecdotal reports of patients who have undergone transplantation in which portal inflow was provided by a large splanchnic collateral [7, 8].

In our patient retrograde dissection to the SMV, thrombectomy, and the use of a donor vein graft provided adequate inflow into the donor portal vein. Her initial postoperative course would indicate that the allograft was well vascularized with both arterial and venous inflow. Thus, one needs to question why this patient developed rethrombosis. In adult recipients, vascular complications are relatively uncommon. Lerut reported a 3.7% incidence of hepatic arterial thrombosis and 1% incidence of portal vein thrombosis in 216 transplants in adults [9]. Portal vein thrombosis has been associated with a number of risk factors including (1) technical factors such as torsion, distal obstruction, or anastomotic stenosis; (2) poor inflow as a result of a preexisting portasystemic shunt, previous splenectomy, previous portal vein injury, or manipulation, large venous collaterals, or a hypoplastic portal vein; (3) hypercoagulable state; (4) preexisting portal vein thrombosis [10]. This patient had several of these risk factors, including a patent DSRS, previous manipulation, and preexisting thrombus in the portal vein and SMV. After extensive laboratory testing which included evaluation for protein S, protein C, and antithrombin III deficiencies, we could not define a primary hypercoagulable state.

Once the diagnosis of posttransplant portal vein thrombosis was made, the patient was returned to the operating room for attempted repair. This decision was based on the degree of allograft dysfunction, the extent of necrosis on biopsy, and the clinical presentation of variceal hemorrhage. In the absence of significant allograft dysfunction or variceal hemorrhage, nonoperative management is reasonable. In our patient, it became apparent from the deterioration in the allograft function that allograft survival would be dependent on adequate splanchnic venous inflow and that variceal hemorrhage would be difficult to manage without portal decompression. Good portal vein flow was reestablished following thrombectomy of the donor portal vein, interposition vein graft, and SMV. Because of our concern for rethrombosis and the fact that she had no inflow from the splenic vein because of the patent DSRS, we elected to provide additional inflow from a large splanchnic venous collateral. This collateral was located along the lesser curvature of the stomach, and with mobilization there was adequate length for direct anastomosis to the donor portal vein. The end-to-side anastomosis was done near the hilum of the liver, distal to the area of thrombosis.

Postoperatively, the hepatic allograft function improved significantly and the patient stopped bleeding from varices. Our major concern at that time was to prevent rethrombosis of the portal venous system. There is no consensus on postoperative management following portal vein thrombectomy and reconstruction. The use of heparin or antiplatelet drugs in the early postoperative period is risky, particularly with a preexisting coagulopathy and hepatic dysfunction. In patients with Budd–Chiari syndrome or a demonstrated hypercoagulable state, anticoagulation is warranted and the risk of bleeding complications accepted. In our patient, it was felt that portal vein rethrombosis would likely be a terminal event from either allograft failure or variceal hemorrhage. Therefore, the patient was treated with a continuous heparin infusion, and liver function and blood counts were carefully monitored. Doppler ultrasonography was utilized to assess arterial and venous inflow into the allograft and patency of the DSRS. The patient was also observed closely for signs of gastrointestinal hemorrhage. After 6 months of heparin therapy (first I.V., then S.Q.) she was converted to warfarin, and anticoagulation continued for 1 year. At that point, antiplatelet therapy was substituted for warfarin. The patient is doing well 2 years posttransplant and has had no allograft dysfunction or recurrent variceal bleeding. Upper endoscopy 1 year posttransplant documented resolution of gastric and esophageal varices.

REFERENCES

1. Langnas AN, Marujo W, Stratta RJ, Wood RP, Shaw BW. Vascular complications after orthotopic liver transplant. *Am J Surg* 1991;161:76–83.
2. AbouJaoude MM, Grant RG, Ghent CN, Mimeault RE, Wall WW. Ef-

fect of portasystemic shunts on subsequent transplantation of the liver. *Surg Gynecol Obstet* 1991;172:215–219.

3. Mazzaferro V, Todo S, Tzakis AG, Stieber A, Makowka L, Starzl TE. Liver transplantation in patients with previous portasystemic shunt. *Am J Surg* 1990;160:111–116.

4. Ring EJ, Lake JR, Roberts JP, Gordon RL, Laberge JM, Read AE, Sterneck MR, Ascher NL. Using transjugular intrahepatic portosystemic shunts to control variceal bleeding before liver transplantation. *Ann Intern Med* 1992;116:304–309.

5. Lind CD, Malisch TW, Chong WK, Richards WO, Pinson CW, Meranze S, Mazer M. Incidence of shunt occlusion or stenosis with transjugular intrahepatic portosystemic shunts (TIPS). *Gastroenterology* 1993;104:A941.

6. Iwatsuki S, Starzl TE, Todo S, Gordon RD, Tzakis AG, March JW, Makowka L, Konero B, Steiber A, Klintmalm G, Husberg B, van Thiel D. Liver transplantation in the treatment of bleeding esophageal varices. *Surgery* 1988;104:697–705.

7. Castaldo P, Langnas AN, Stratta RJ, Lieberman RP, Wood RP, Shaw BW. Successful liver transplantation in a patient with a thrombosed portomestenteric system after multiple failed shunts. *Am J Gastroenterol* 1991;86:506–508.

8. Hiatt JR, Quinones-Baldrich WJ, Ramming KP, Lois JF, Busuttil RW. Bile duct varices. An alternative to portoportal anastomosis in liver transplantation. *Transplantation* 1986;42:85.

9. Lerut JP, Gordon RD, Iwatsuki S, Starzl TE. Human orthotopic liver transplantation. Surgical aspects in 393 consecutive grafts. *Transplant Proceed* 1988;20:603–606.

10. Lerut JP, Tzakis AG, Bron K, Gordon RD, Iwatsuki S, Esquivel C, Makowka L, Todo S, Starzl TE. Complications of venous reconstruction in human OLTX. *Ann Surg* 1987;205:404–414.

19

Decreased Vision in a Liver Transplant Candidate

James G. Drougas, David S. Raiford, and C. Wright Pinson

CLINICAL PRESENTATION

History of Present Illness

A 45-year-old man with a long-standing history of ulcerative colitis and primary sclerosing cholangitis was referred to our facility for evaluation for orthotopic liver transplantation. The patient presented initially at age 30, with an 8-year history of intermittent diarrhea that was occasionally bloody. The diagnosis of ulcerative colitis was confirmed with colonoscopy. The patient was managed medically with control of his symptoms until age 40, at which time he developed recurrent bloody diarrhea and was found to have elevated hepatic biochemical tests.

Over the next 4 years the patient's liver dysfunction worsened. This was manifested biochemically by a progressive rise in his serum bilirubin to a peak of 15 mg/dl, an alkaline phosphatase of 1800 IU/L, a serum albumin of 2.9 mg/dl, and a prothrombin time of 15 s. Clinical manifestations of hepatic dysfunction included frequent episodes of epistaxis and intractable pruritus, despite treatment with cholestyramine. He denied bone pain. A percutaneous liver biopsy revealed cirrhosis with cholestasis, and contrast study of the biliary system was consistent with primary sclerosing cholangitis. He required hospitalization on one occasion for an episode of acute cholangitis. Due to the duration of his colitis, surveillance colonoscopy was performed, and biopsies revealed moderate dysplasia of the left colon. Total abdominal colectomy with ileostomy was performed in anticipation of liver transplantation. No frank malignancy was identified in the resected colon. Two months before transplantation, the patient noted the insidious onset of decreased visual acuity, especially at night, xerophthalmia, and a yellow hue to his vision.

Physical Exam

The patient's exam was remarkable for scleral icterus, normal funduscopic exam, and mild jaundice. There was no palpable lymphadenopathy or abdominal masses. There was no organomegaly and he had no stigmata of portal hypertension. His midline incision was healing well and his ileostomy was patent.

Laboratory Data

The results of laboratory tests were the following:

Electrolytes	normal
Glucose	90 mg/dl
Creatinine	0.6 mg/dl
BUN	8 mg/dl
Bilirubin	5.2 mg/dl
SGOT	51 IU/L
LDH	232 IU/L
Alkaline phosphatase	620 IU/L
Albumin	2.8 g/dl
PT	15 s
PTT	38 s
PCV	39%
WBC	7,400/mm^3
Serum vitamin A	6 μg/dl (normal, 24–106 μg/dl)
25-hydroxyvitamin D$_3$	7 ng/ml (normal, 16–74 ng/ml)

COURSE

The patient was given water-miscible retinol palmitate (Aquasol A) 50,000 units/day intramuscularly for 3 days, followed by 25,000 units/day orally for 1 week. Vitamin D replacement therapy was initiated with 1,25-

dihydroxyvitamin D_3 (Rocaltrol) 0.25 μg/day orally. He noticed improvement in his vision within 24 h and normalization within 1 week of treatment. Orthotopic liver transplantation was accomplished 10 weeks after his total abdominal colectomy.

DIAGNOSIS

The diagnosis was hypovitaminosis A.

DISCUSSION

The fat-soluble vitamins A, D, and K play vital roles in metabolism and hemostasis. Although hypovitaminosis of the fat-soluble vitamins was a significant medical problem in the past and remains so today in developing countries, few patients develop fat-soluble hypovitaminosis due to dietary insufficiency. Proper absorption of these vitamins hinges upon adequate delivery of bile salts into the intestine, which promotes absorption of dietary fat. Some patients with advanced liver disease may be unable to excrete bile salts in amounts adequate to enable proper absorption of dietary fats; this can lead to fat-soluble hypovitaminosis.

Bile salt are metabolites of cholesterol. The adult liver synthesizes between 200–600 mg/day of bile salts and secretes between 12–36 g/day of bile salts into the small bowel; 95% of which is recovered via the enterohepatic circulation. Bile salts aid in fat digestion in two ways. First, they facilitate hydrolysis of acylglycerols into fatty acids. Second, they form micelles which enhance mucosal surface contact of hydrophobic compounds, thus facilitating transport across the intestinal brush border into the enterocyte, then into the lymphatic system as chylomicrons or directly into the portal circulation. Any disease process that interferes with the production of bile acids or their delivery to the intestine can cause fat malabsorption, and thus lead to inadequate absorption of the fat-soluble vitamins. Of note, treatment of pruritus with bile salt binding resins such as cholestyramine may worsen malabsorption by decreasing further the availability of bile acids within the intestinal lumen.

Vitamin A

Man's interest in vitamin A dates back thousands of years when the Egyptians realized night blindness could be cured by eating animal liver

[1]. However, it was not until 1915 that McCallum and Davis first described a fat-soluble factor which was growth-promoting. Drummond later coined the term vitamin A, and George Wald was awarded the Nobel Prize for Medicine in 1967 for elucidating the role of vitamin A in the visual system.

The term vitamin A refers to several biologically active compounds: retinol (vitamin A_1), 3-dehydroretinol (vitamin A_2), and the ester forms of vitamin A_1 or A_2. Over 90% of the total body reserve of vitamin A is stored in the ester form within the liver. Retinal is the aldehyde form of retinol and it is the active form of vitamin A in vision. The carotenoids, which include alpha-, beta-, and gamma-carotene and lycopene, are structurally similar to vitamin A and considered provitamins.

Dietary vitamin A derives almost exclusively from animal sources. Animal and fish liver have the highest concentration of vitamin A, whereas other significant sources include milk products and eggs. Provitamin A, the carotenoids, occur in plants such as soybean and fruits. Provitamin A is converted to vitamin A within the intestinal wall in humans, whereas vitamin A itself is absorbed directly from the small intestine. The all-trans retinyl ester comprises the major dietary form of vitamin A. This form is hydrolyzed within the intestine, absorbed in a micellar form, incorporated into chylomicrons, and transported to the systemic circulation via the thoracic duct. It is subsequently stored in the liver as retinyl ester and transported to target tissues in a complex that consists of one molecule retinol, one prealbumin molecule, and one molecule of retinol-binding protein (RBP). It is important to note that the serum level of vitamin A (normal, 24–106 µg/dl) is preserved until hepatic stores are exhausted; thus, a patient with a normal serum level may have critically low reserves. Repeated studies have shown that the most accurate means of assessing vitamin A deficiency is by quantitative analysis of liver tissue obtained on biopsy, although this is seldom done in clinical practice.

The function of vitamin A within the visual system is complex. Whereas cones are concerned primarily with color vision, rods are associated with vision in dim light. Vitamin A is involved in both systems in conjunction with two different proteins. In rod cells, retinal combines with the protein opsin, forming the photosensitive pigment rhodopsin. When a quantum of light is absorbed by rhodopsin, the retinal is isomerized and produces nervous excitation that is transmitted to the brain via the optic nerve. In addition to its incorporation into visual pigment, vitamin A promotes epithelial integrity and maintains differentiation of epithelial surfaces. Furthermore, vitamin A probably assists in the maintenance of host resistance to bacterial infection, although the mechanisms accounting for this are not established. Animals deprived of vitamin A will eventually die.

The initial symptom of hypovitaminosis A is night blindness (nyctalopia), which is due to the lack of retinal with which to form rhodopsin. This condition is fully reversible with dietary supplementation. However, xerophthalmia (drying of the cornea) also occurs and can progress to corneal ulceration and perforation. This xerosis can also occur throughout the body with keratinization of columnar epithelium and pathologic calcification. Structural deformity of the cornea may lead to irreversible blindness. Thus, permanent visual loss due to hypovitaminosis A results from deficits in maintenance of corneal integrity rather than from inability to form adequate visual pigment.

Our patient presented with classic symptoms of night blindness and dry eyes. The onset of these symptoms was insidious. He was predisposed to fat-soluble hypovitaminosis due to his advanced cholestatic liver. Treatment of patients with ocular findings consists of parenteral then oral vitamin A replacement. Thus, our patient received a total of 150,000 units of water-miscible retinol palmitate (Aquasol A) given parenterally over 3 days followed by 25,000 units/day orally for 1 week. Because vitamin A stores in normal adult liver are approximately 500,000 units, up to half of this amount may be given over several days by intramuscular injection and then the balance of replacement given orally. For patients at high risk for deficiency due to malabsorption or cholestyramine therapy, prophylaxis may be given by administering 25,000 units orally twice weekly [2]. As the liver is the site of vitamin A storage, hepatic replacement is curative, and supplementation posttransplantation generally unnecessary.

Vitamin D

Two types of osteodystrophy complicate chronic liver disease. Osteoporosis is a multifactorial disorder which entails proportionate reduction in bone mineral and protein matrix. In contrast, osteomalacia is almost invariably due to vitamin D deficiency and is characterized by bone loss with a mineralization deficit and a relative excess of uncalcified protein matrix. The disease process of softening of bones was recognized several hundred years ago and termed rickets. Today, it is known that rickets occurs when newly formed bone matrix fails to mineralize. In 1807, Bardsley recognized that cod liver oil was efficacious in the treatment of osteomalacia, while in 1922, Sir Edward Mellanby found he could prevent rickets in animals treated with cod liver oil. McCollum termed this factor vitamin D in the early part of this century.

The D vitamins are sterols that have a triene structure [3]. The active forms of the compound can be generated within the dermis in the presence of ultraviolet light which converts ergosterol to ergocalciferol (vitamin D_2) and 7-dehydrocholesterol to cholecalciferol (vitamin D_3). Vitamin D is also classified as a hormone as it undergoes feedback inhibition of its synthesis. As with the other fat-soluble vitamins, vitamin D is absorbed with fat; thus, underlying liver disease that decreases bile acid delivery or production can cause its malabsorption. It is absorbed from the small bowel and is transported within chylomicrons via the lymphatics to the liver. There it is hydroxylated to form 25-hydroxyvitamin D_3, the most predominant form in man. Subsequent 1-hydroxylation within the kidney results in the bioactive metabolite 1,25-dihydroxyvitamin D_3.

Vitamin D facilitates mineralization of bone and endochondral calcification. In so doing, it prevents rickets in children and osteomalacia in adults. It also maintains calcium homeostasis. A fall in the serum calcium concentration stimulates the secretion of parathormone, which, in turn, stimulates the synthesis of 1,25-dihydroxyvitamin D_3 in the kidney. This active vitamin D_3 metabolite stimulates the absorption of intestinal calcium and phosphorus and, together with parathormone, enhances renal reabsorption of calcium and mobilization of calcium from bone. Once the serum calcium level is restored to normal, parathormone release is suppressed and, thus, the rate of synthesis of 1,25-dihydroxyvitamin D_3 is decreased. The mechanism of action of 1,25-dihydroxyvitamin D_3 is receptor mediated. After binding to a cytosolic receptor, this complex is transported to the nucleus where it initiates transcription of genes coding for calcium and phosphate transport proteins.

The etiology of hepatic osteodystrophy is multifactorial and contributants may include hypovitaminosis D, hypogonadism, tobacco abuse, alcohol abuse, and calcium malnutrition. In addition, some patients require corticosteroids prior to transplantation, which may worsen their bone disease, and all of these patients will be on corticosteroids following transplantation. The clinical consequence of hypovitaminosis D is osteomalacia, which may complicate osteoporosis. Hepatic osteodystrophy may be quite debilitating for patients with advanced cholestatic liver disease [4–8]. These patients are prone to bone pain, kyphosis, and spontaneous compression fractures of the vertebrae. Thus, detecting osteopenia early in the course of disease may help conserve bone density prior to liver replacement.

Serum levels of 25-hydroxyvitamin D_3 and 1,25-dihydroxyvitamin D_3 can be measured and reflect adequacy of vitamin D nutriture; yet they do not correlate well with the severity of bone disease. This patient had a 25-hydroxyvitamin D_3 level prior to transplantation of 6 μg/dl (normal, 24–106 μg/dl) and treatment was initiated prior to liver transplantation. It is important to recognize that although Vitamin D replacement is effective in the treatment of osteomalacia, it may not be helpful in the prevention or treatment of osteoporosis.

Established hypovitaminosis D or biopsy proved osteomalacia can be treated with oral replacement as vitamin D_2 (ergocalciferol) 50,000 units/day, vitamin D_3 (cholecalciferol) 4000 units/day, or 1,25-dihydroxyvitamin D_3, 0.25 μg/day. None of these agents should be administered within 2 h of cholestyramine. Replacement therapy over several months may be necessary to restore vitamin D nutriture. Prophylactic vitamin D therapy can be given in identical doses twice weekly. As hypervitaminosis D may cause appreciable toxicity and there is no evidence that supplementation affects the risk for osteoporosis, routine administration of vitamin D is discouraged. Those patients receiving long-term supplementation should be monitored periodically for hypercalcemia and hyperphosphatemia. From a practical perspective, the safest way for patients with cholestasis to avoid hypovitaminosis D is to promote cutaneous vitamin D synthesis by exposing skin to direct sunlight for 15–20 min daily.

Vitamin K

Vitamin K was the last fat-soluble vitamin to be identified. In 1929, Dam identified a hemorrhagic disease in chicks fed a fat-extracted diet. He subsequently identified a substance that played a role in coagulation and termed it vitamin K, for Koagulation vitamin. It was later found that the anticoagulant effect of vitamin K deficiency was produced by a reduction in the content of plasma prothrombin (factor II) and factors VII, IX, and X. A form of vitamin K was isolated from plants, phylloquinone (K_1), and a form was identified in fishmeal, menaquinone (K_2). Dietary sources for vitamin K include green leafy vegetables; yet, the vitamin is also synthesized by endogenous intestinal flora. Of the fat-soluble vitamins, vitamin K is the most dependent on luminal bile salts for its proper absorption.

Vitamin K functions as a cofactor in the coagulation cascade. It is involved in the enzymatic alp-carboxylation of glutamic acid residues on factors II, VII, IX, and X. This carboxylation converts these proteins to their active form by enabling them to bind calcium during thrombogenesis. Without γ-carboxylation, these factors are hypofunctional and, thus, the prothrombin time is prolonged. The normal liver has a 30-day store of vitamin K, but this is decreased in patients with underlying liver disease and can be rapidly depleted. Due to its short serum half-life of 6 h, factor VII appears to be depleted first, followed by factors II and X, and then factor IX.

This patient had a mildly elevated prothrombin time and experienced episodes of epistaxis. Contributants to coagulopathy in this setting may include a global decrease synthesis of clotting proteins, accelerated fibrinolysis, and decreased absorption of vitamin K. In patients with end-stage liver disease or biliary obstruction, treatment with subcutaneous vitamin K (Aquamephyton) 10 mg daily for 3 days may improve the prothrombin time and improve hemostasis. If prolongation of the prothrombin time is due to vitamin K deficiency, improvement may be seen as soon as 8 h after a dose of parenteral vitamin K.

Prophylaxis against recurrent vitamin K deficiency may be given orally as phytonadione (Mephyton) 5–10 mg daily. Because vitamin K absorption is crucially dependent on bile acids, it may be advantageous to consider concomitant oral administration of the hydrophilic bile salt ursodiol (Actigall) 300 mg. This may enhance absorption in patients who respond to parenteral vitamin K but who appear to malabsorb oral replacement. Neither of these agents should be given within 2 h of cholestyramine.

CONCLUSION

Management of patients with end-stage liver disease presents many problems for clinicians. Patients with end-stage cholestatic liver disease are at high risk for fat-soluble vitamin deficiency on the basis of malabsorption [1]. Although vitamin K deficiency appears to be the most commonly recognized deficiency, hypovitaminosis A and D occur often in patients whose cholestatic liver disease is severe enough to warrant consideration of transplantation. The patient presented developed debilitating night blindness as well as corneal xerosis and had biochemical evidence of hypovitaminosis D. If unrecognized, remediable impairments in blood clotting, mucosal integrity, and bone strength can contribute significantly to peritransplant morbidity. We feel that all patients with cholestatic liver disease for whom transplantation is being considered should be screened for fat-soluble hypovitaminosis. Those patients who are at increased risk for (e.g., those receiving cholestyramine) or with documented deficiency states should receive vitamin supplements until transplantation is accomplished, as hepatic replacement is usually curative.

REFERENCES

1. Bikle D. Metabolism and functions of Vitamins A,D, and K. In *Physiology and Biochemistry of Normal Hepatic Function.* 182–186.
2. Amedee-Manesme O, Furr H, Alvarez F, Hadshouel M, Alagille D, Olson J. Biochemical indicators of vitamin A depletion in children with cholestasis. *Hepatology* 1985;6:1143–1182.
3. DeLuca H. Vitamin D. In: *The Foundations of Nutrition.* 160–169.
4. Rabinovitv M, Shapiro J, Lian J, Block G, Merkel I, Van Thiel D. Vitamin D and osteocalcin levels in liver transplant recipients; Is osteocalcin a reliable marker of bone turnover in such cases? *J Hepatol* 1992;16:50–55.
5. Guanabens N, Pares A, Marinoso L, Brancos M, Piera C, Serrano S, Rivera F, Rodes J. Factors influencing the development of metabolic bone disease in primary biliary cirrhosis. *Am J Gastroenterol* 1990;85:1356–1362.
6. Floreani A, Chiaramonte M, Giannini S, Malvasi L, Lodetti M, Castignano R, Giacomini A, D'Angelo A, Naccarato R. Longitudinal study on osteodystrophy in primary biliary cirrhosis and a pilot study on calcitonin treatment. *J Hepatol* 1991;12:217–223.
7. Compston J. Hepatic osteodystrophy: Vitamin D metabolism in patients with liver disease. *Gut* 1986;27:1073–1090.
8. Kaplan M, Elta G, Furie B, Sadowski J, Russell R. Fat-soluble vitamin nutriture in primary biliary cirrhosis. *Gastroenterology*, 1988;95:787–792.

20

New Treatment Options for Liver Failure

James G. Drougas and J. Kelly Wright, Jr.

CLINICAL PRESENTATION

History

A 34-year-old man was referred to our institution for evaluation and management of massive hemorrhage from esophageal varices. He initially presented 2 weeks earlier to an another hospital with hematemesis and shock. During his resuscitation he received 30 units of packed red blood cells, fresh frozen plasma, vasopressin, and dopamine to restore his blood pressure. Emergent esophagogastroduodenoscopy (EGD) revealed large bleeding esophageal varices that were sclerosed. No further bleeding was noted. His prothrombin time on admission was 28.6 and improved to 18 with transfusion of fresh frozen plasma. His serum bilirubin rose from 2.2 mg/dl at presentation to 12.7 mg/dl at the time of transfer to our medical center.

His past medical history was remarkable for alcohol abuse since the age of 19 and an intermittent history of intravenous drug use. Despite two prior attempts at alcohol rehabilitation, the patient had been drinking heavily at the time of this admission. Although alcoholic liver disease had been documented for several years, he began to have manifestations of portal hypertension with two previous variceal bleeds only within the past year. Sclerotherapy had been performed on five sepa-

rate occasions due to his recurrent bleeding. He had undergone ton-
sillectomy and inguinal herniorrhaphy as a child. His medicines at the
time of transfer to our hospital included prilosec 20 mg qd, spirono-
lactone 50 mg bid, sucralfate 1 g qid and lactulose 30 cc tid. His family
history was notable for an uncle and grandfather who suffered from
alcoholism.

On referral, the patient was hemodynamically stable. He was not or-
thostatic and had no stigmata of hepatic encephalopathy. He had moderate scleral icterus and numerous spider angiomata over his chest and
back. His abdomen was soft and not tender with mild hepatomegaly,
no splenomegaly, and moderate ascites. Upon rectal exam he was found
to have external hemorrhoids and occult blood in his stool.

Laboratory Data

The results of laboratory tests were as follows:

	2/28/91	3/19/91
Electrolytes	normal	normal
Glucose	85 mg/dl	90 mg/dl
Creatinine	0.7 mg/dl	0.8 mg/dl
BUN	12 mg/dl	10 mg/dl
Bilirubin	2.2 mg/dl	12.7 mg/dl
SGOT		51 IU/L
LDH		232 IU/L
Alkaline phosphatase		101 IU/L
Ammonia		36 mg/L
Albumin	1.3 g/dl	2.6 g/dl
Fibrinogen		105 mg/dl
PT	28.6 s	17 s
PTT		38 s
PCV	16%	30%
WBC	6060/cc	4700/cc

Hospital Course

The patient was identified as a having Child–Pugh class C cirrhosis
(12/15 points) and unreformed alcoholism. Although significant hepatic synthetic dysfunction existed, the portal hypertension and recurrent hemorrhage were the major clinical issues in need of control. Pan-

hepatic arteriography and wedged hepatic venography revealed grade II hepatopetal flow, normal anatomy of the portal venous system, and corrected sinusoidal pressure of 23 mm Hg. Endoscopy demonstrated moderate-sized esophageal varices with sclerotherapy-induced erosions in the distal esophagus. There was no evidence of active bleeding. Intensive alcohol abuse counseling was begun along with vitamin, mineral, and nutritional supplementation.

On the sixth day of his hospitalization, the patient vomited 1700 cc of bloody emesis. Emergent EGD demonstrated oozing varices. Bleeding continued despite sclerotherapy and intravenous vasopressin. A Sengstaken–Blakemore tube was placed which temporarily controlled the hemorrhage. Transhepatic splenoportagraphy was performed, which demonstrated extensive short gastric varices and a large left gastric varix. The mean portal pressure was 35 mm Hg. These gastric varices and the coronary vein were individually embolized with Gelfoam and Gianturco coils with cessation of the variceal bleeding.

Two days after transhepatic embolization, recurrent bleeding was suspected. Repeat EGD showed no actively bleeding varices; however, there was blood streaming from the ampulla of Vater. The hemobilia was due to injury of an aberrant right hepatic artery at the time of transhepatic splenoportagraphy. The patient was returned to the radiology suite where coil embolization of the distal right hepatic artery was performed. Although his bleeding was controlled transiently, progressive hepatic failure was noted with worsening coagulopathy, encephalopathy, and jaundice.

He was enrolled in an experimental protocol utilizing an artificial liver support system using a bioartificial liver (BAL) with porcine hepatocytes. A double lumen hemodialysis catheter was placed in his superficial femoral vein and the patient was connected to a standard plasmapheresis circuit into which the hepatocyte reactor was added. The patient underwent a single 6-h treatment with the BAL. He remained hemodynamically stable during the pheresis. Although there was only a slight improvement in his mental status, his coagulation factors increased and his ammonia level dropped measurably, as illustrated in Fig. 20-1. With ongoing general medical supportive care. The patient's condition gradually improved.

Because of intermittent oozing from portal gastropathy and esophageal ulcerations, he was considered for a new nonsurgical portal decompressive procedure with placement of a transjugular intrahepatic portosystemic shunt (TIPS). A 10-mm Wall stent was placed between the right branch of the portal vein and the right hepatic vein. Portography revealed numerous new gastric varices that had developed since

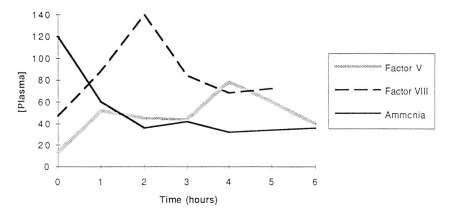

Figure 20-1. Biochemical and hepatic function markers during artificial liver support.

previous transhepatic embolization. After construction of the TIPS, the portal pressure was reduced to 20 mm Hg from 34 mm Hg. No further bleeding was noted, and his clinical course gradually improved.

A color flow Doppler ultrasonogram 6 weeks after discharge showed a patent TIPS with a flow velocity of 78 cm/s. EGD revealed resolution of his esophageal varices and only mild portal hypertensive gastropathy. Subsequently, a shuntogram was obtained to measure the pressure gradient across the TIPS. The splenic and portal pressures were 27 mm Hg each. The pressure in the middle of the shunt was 27 mm Hg, whereas the hepatic venous and inferior vena caval pressures were 14 and 13 mm Hg, respectively. Over the next several months the patient continued to abstain from alcohol. He completed an inpatient alcohol rehabilitation program, which was followed by an aggressive outpatient therapy. Biochemical profile revealed an hematocrit of 31%, prothrombin time of 18 s, albumin of 3.1 g/dl, and a bilirubin of 7.4 mg/dl. Seven months after discharge, the patient underwent orthotopic liver transplantation. The explanted native liver demonstrated diffuse micronodular cirrhosis and a patent TIPS with slight intimal hyperplasia on the hepatic vein side of the shunt; its internal diameter was 10 mm at the portal vein and 5 mm at the hepatic vein. His posttransplant recovery was uneventful. The patient is now over a year after transplantation and he is back at work as a safety supervisor in an industrial construction job.

DISCUSSION

Liver failure remains a major cause of mortality in the United States. Over 27,000 people died in 1990 from liver failure. Although orthotopic liver transplantation (OLT) has become the ideal treatment for end-stage liver disease, not all patients are candidates for this procedure. Contraindications for OLT include sepsis, metastatic neoplasia, advanced age, co-morbid cardiorespiratory insufficiency, AIDS, and active alcoholism or substance abuse. For patients actively listed for OLT, approximately 25% die of progressive liver failure while awaiting their transplants due to a widespread shortage of donor organs.

Beyond liver replacement, the mainstay of care for patients with end-stage liver disease is supportive. However, two recent technological advances may prove to expand the therapeutic options available for patients with hepatic failure and its numerous sequelae. As noted for the patient in the case presentation, aggressive and intensive medical support did not provide clinical stabilization until his portal hypertension was controlled and acute reversible hepatic dysfunction was resolved. Although measurable improvements in the patient's biochemical profile were noted during the application of the BAL, the therapeutic benefit of BAL for this patient was of less significance than establishing the safety of this technology in human subjects. In the future, artificial liver support systems like the BAL may offer a potential bridge to OLT or allow liver regeneration following an acute injury. For the management of end-stage liver disease and variceal hemorrhage, TIPS potentially can provide decompression of portal hypertension, control bleeding, and stabilize critically ill patients.

BIOARTIFICIAL LIVER FOR HEPATIC FAILURE

The feasibility of an artificial liver support system has been studied for the past 35 years. Early work attempted to control hepatic encephalopathy by diluting or adsorbing circulating toxins with hemodialysis, charcoal column hemoperfusion, or exchange transfusions. Although transient mild improvement in encephalopathy was noted, no improvement in patient survival from hepatic failure was demonstrated. Although the liver plays a vital role in detoxification, this is only one of numerous metabolic functions with which the liver is involved. The liver also synthesizes several plasma proteins, stores glycogen, and performs numerous biotransformations. With the complexity of the metabolic and physiologic functions of the liver requiring support in an anhepatic patient, a better model for artificial liver support requires viable hepatic tissue mass.

The next phase of investigation into an artificial liver support system studied closed-system perfusion of functioning exogenous hepatocytes with either homologous (other human) or heterologous (other species) livers. The first use of a human cadaveric liver for extracorporeal perfusion was reported by Sen et al. in 1966 [1]. They demonstrated a significant improvement in the patients' biochemical parameters, but patient survival was unchanged. Whereas the current use of human livers is reserved for OLT, the study of extracorporeal perfusion of xenografts continues, although preformed natural antibodies prevent the use of some species combinations. At this time, the long-term immunologic sequelae of ex vivo whole organ hepatic perfusion remain unclear.

More recent advances in the development of an artificial liver system involve the use of harvested or cultured hepatocytes supported on a synthetic framework. These systems have been designed either to be implanted or to be perfused extracorporeally. Initial work on the BAL used free cultured hepatocytes harvested from either pigs or dogs. However, under standard cell-culture conditions, normal hepatocytes lose their tissue-specific functions in 3–5 days and the cells die within 1–2 weeks. Although hepatocytes transformed by viruses and neoplasia have less stringent growth requirements, their clinical application remains unclear due to unknown potential for disease transmission to the recipient. Nontransformed, cultured hepatocyte survival, and differentiated function was greatly improved as the use of special culture media, mitogens, growth factors, and extracellular matrices were developed [2].

An implantable BAL was first described by Matas et al. when they used free hepatocyte transplantation for the potential treatment of metabolic deficiencies in rats in 1976 [3]. Further work by Demetriou et al. has shown that these liver xenocytes attached to microcarriers have better engraftment in the recipient and can synthesize albumin and conjugate bilirubin if injected intraportally or into the peritoneal cavity [4]. The transplanted hepatocytes also can be enclosed within alginate-collagen gel microdroplets; microencapsulation allows diffusion of nutrients to the hepatocytes and diffusion of synthetic products away from the cells. This technique provides an immunologic barrier between the transplanted cells and the recipient, as molecular and cellular interactions with antibodies and lymphocytes cannot cross this barrier. These microencapsulated hepatocytes have been shown to conjugate bile and prolong survival in an animal model of fulminant hepatic failure without the need for immunosuppression.

Although the implantable BAL remains untested in humans, extracorporeal BAL devices have been tested clinically. Investigations with "hepatodialysis" (dialysis against an diffusion bioreactor with an hepa-

tocyte suspension) for the management of acute liver failure were reported in the late 1980s [5]. Modest improvements in survival were noted,
although comparison groups were poorly matched.

Further advances have led to the hollow-fiber cartridge bioreactor,
which consists of normal hepatocytes attached to a microcarrier gel placed
on the extracapillary side of the bioreactor (Fig. 20-2). The semiperme-
able cellulose acetate fibers of the bioreactor have a nominal molecular
weight cutoff of 70,000 daltons, which is large enough to allow diffusion of small molecules and many hepatic synthetic proteins; however
cellular material and immunoglobulins are excluded. The hepatocytes
perform both synthetic and metabolic functions and the by-products
diffuse back across the fibers into the intracapillary space. Cultured hepatocytes, when attached to microcarriers, will synthesize albumin and
clotting factors, conjugate bilirubin, and perform numerous metabolic
functions normally performed by the liver. Scattered clinical reports

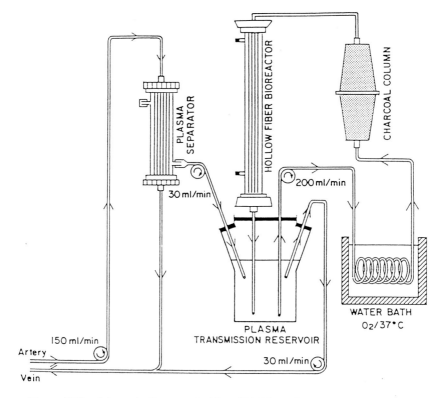

Figure 20-2. Schematic diagram of a bioartificial liver (BAL) support system. (From
Ref. 6.)

suggest the minimal mass of hepatic tissue in the bioreactor be 10% of the recipient's native liver [6].

The BAL has made tremendous advances over the past 10 years. Both the implantable and the extracorporeal liver support systems use functioning xenograft hepatocytes that can perform the numerous complex functions of the normal liver. The current advantages of the extracorporeal system include the avoidance of immunosuppressive medications, the immediate availability of a bioreactor with xenograft harvesting techniques, and the system can be recharged with viable hepatocytes as needed. Despite these advances, problems such as optimum hepatocyte mass requirement and immunologic sequelae have yet to be resolved. The current use of the BAL remains an extraordinary research measure for patients with liver failure for whom an immediate hepatic transplantation is not available.

TIPS FOR UNCONTROLLED PORTAL HYPERTENSION

The management of patients with recurrent or severe variceal hemorrhage has undergone considerable evolution. Endoscopic sclerotherapy has become the initial treatment for active bleeding. Acute variceal hemorrhage can be acutely controlled with sclerotherapy 80% of the time, but the recurrence of variceal hemorrhage is unfortunately high. Those patients who fail sclerotherapy should be considered for decompression by portosystemic shunting or for liver transplantation, yet shortage of donor liver allografts often precludes immediate liver replacement. Emergent central portosystemic shunt (portocaval, mesocaval, central splenorenal shunts) remains a major surgical procedure accompanied by significant morbidity and mortality in debilitated patients with minimal hepatic functional reserve. Despite aggressive treatment by either surgical shunting or sclerotherapy, the overall 1-year survival of Child–Pugh Class C cirrhotics is less than 50% with recurrent variceal bleeding accounting for a majority of the morbidity and mortality. Liver transplantation in the face of previous central portosystemic surgical shunt, while feasible, becomes a more formidable and complicated procedure [7]. Control of portal hypertension without major surgical intervention is very appealing, and the development of a percutaneously created portosystemic shunt has followed.

The first successful nonsurgical approach to portosystemic shunting was performed by Jose F. Rosch in 1969 [8]. He percutaneously created a tract through the hepatic parenchyma between the inferior vena cava and portal vein in a swine model. In 1982, Colapinto described a technique of successive balloon dilatations of a parenchymal tract between the portal and hepatic veins in human subjects [9]. However, he demonstrated a patent shunt at 6 months in only 2 of 15 patients treated emergently for bleeding varices. Further refinement of the transjugular intrahepatic portosystemic shunt (TIPS) with the technology of intravascular metal stents has resulted in improved shunt patency and function (Fig. 20-3).

Early clinical reports suggested that the TIPS procedure was relatively safe and effective. Until 1992, small series of TIPS procedures were reported by several centers. Recently, La berge et al. reported their results in 100 patients [10]. Successful shunt placement was achieved 96% of the time. On average, portal pressure was reduced by 10 mm Hg and residual portal–hepatic venous pressure gradient was 10.5 mm Hg. Hemorrhage control was achieved in greater than 90% of patients with bleeding varices, and significant improvement in ascites manage-

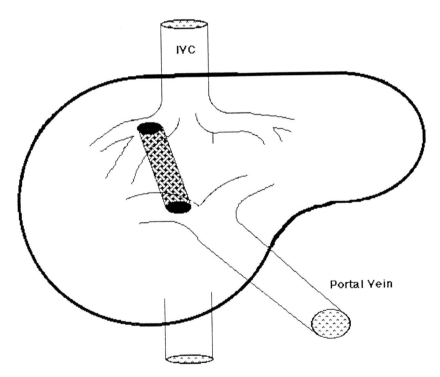

Figure 20-3. Schematic diagram of a transjugular intrahepatic portesystemic shunt (TIPS) with an expandable wire mesh stent bridging the portal venous system to the hepatic veins.

ment was noted in 80%. New onset or worsening of encephalopathy occurred in 18% of patients. Hepatic decompensation after TIPS was noted in 25% of patients as a rise in serum bilirubin. Nine patients died of progressive liver failure within 90 days of TIPS placement, although the role of portal venous shunting in these patients is not clearly defined. Direct TIPS-induced complications were uncommon, but intraperitoneal bleeding, hemobilia, bacteremias, and transient renal failure were noted in small numbers of patients. After an average follow-up of 5 months, shunt stenosis or occlusion was noted in 10% of patients.

Many patients with advanced liver disease complicated by uncontrolled variceal hemorrhage can be optimally managed with orthotopic liver transplantation; however, due to the shortage of donor allografts, emergency hepatic transplantation for variceal bleeding is not always readily available. The technical difficulty of liver transplantation and operative blood loss are greatly increased in patients who have had prior surgical portosystemic shunts or other surgery in the porta hepatis. A recent prospective study addressed the role of TIPS in controlling bleeding from esophageal varices in patients awaiting liver transplantation [11]. Thirteen patients with either active variceal bleeding or recurrent variceal bleeding despite sclerotherapy were treated with TIPS placement. Portal decompression similar to that seen with 8- and 10-mm mesocaval H-grafts was noted. All six patients with active variceal hemorrhage stopped bleeding immediately after successful TIPS placement. One of the 13 developed recurrent variceal bleeding and this was due to shunt occlusion. Seven patients were subsequently transplanted with success. Thus, TIPS may be able to play an important role as a bridge to transplantation by controlling variceal hemorrhage while a suitable hepatic allograft is sought. Other centers have proposed that pretransplantation TIPS placement may facilitate the liver transplantation procedure by controlling portal hypertension and minimizing operative blood loss. TIPS metallic stents undergo intimal incorporation after placement and, therefore, require accurate deployment to prevent compromise of the portal vein and suprahepatic inferior vena cava vascular control and manipulation at liver transplantation [12].

In cirrhotic patients who are not transplant candidates due to a variety of contraindications. TIPS placement has been applied with some success. For the Child's Class C cirrhotic patient where chronic variceal sclerotherapy and portosystemic shunt surgery are accompanied by considerable morbidity. TIPS has provided prompt control of portal hypertension where endoscopy also demonstrates complete variceal decompression in all successfully treated with TIPS. Our patient also had complete decompression of his esophageal varices and a marked reduction in his portal gastropathy after successful portal decompression with TIPS.

Although the work of Palmez et al. demonstrated that long-term patency could be achieved in a canine model [13], the long-term efficacy of TIPS in humans has yet to be determined. Although technological advances with the use of metal stenting make long-term patency more likely, neointimal hyperplasia appears to be a common occurrence in the shunt and ultimately leads to shunt narrowing. Some centers note a TIPS stenosis rate as high as 40% by 5 months [14], and shunt patency rates for 1 year and beyond are not yet reported in large series. Our patient's TIPS had a 50% reduction in diameter at the hepatic vein side after 7 months without clinically significant portal hypertension. For shunt stenosis associated with a concomitant increase in portal pressure, percutaneous balloon angioplasty is one method of salvage. Upon placement of a guide wire across the stent, the primary shunt can be dilated or a second stent can be placed within the old one and then expanded. Color doppler sonography offers a noninvasive outpatient technique for evaluating shunt function. Sonography can demonstrate shunt diameter, shunt patency, and flow velocity.

The long-term benefit of TIPS placement is by no means certain. However, at this time, the evolving data seem to suggest that it is a safe and efficacious procedure in selected settings. TIPS can act as a bridge to hepatic transplantation. It may allow stabilization of the patient with refractory variceal bleeding in order that a proper pretransplant evaluation and allograft retrieval be completed. TIPS is effective in treating those nontransplant candidates who are at extremely high risk for surgical shunting and can provide a safer method for control of variceal bleeding in the patient with decompensated liver failure. However younger patients with a good hepatic reserve may be better served with a selective surgical shunt that has excellent long-term patency, as early reports for TIPS suggest less durability and questionable long-term shunt patency.

CONCLUSION

Patients with acute liver failure and end-stage liver disease remain among the most challenging groups of patients to manage clinically. There are few effective treatment options to support these patients' liver function, especially during episodes of potentially reversible complications (variceal hemorrhage, sepsis, encephalopathy). Artificial liver support systems and TIPS offer the clinician an expanded arsenal to manage liver failure or to support a patient to liver replacement through transplantation.

REFERENCES

1. Sen PK, Bhalerao RA, Parulkar GP, Samsi AB, Shah BK, Kinare SG. Use of isolated perfused cadaveric liver in the management of hepatic failure. *Surgery* 1966;59:774–781.
2. Nyberg SL, Shatford RA, Wei-shou H, Payne WD, Cerra FB. Hepatocyte culture systems for artificial liver support. *Crit Care Med* 1992;20:1157–1168.
3. Matas AJ, Sutherland DE, Steffes MW, Mauer SM, Sowe A, Simmons RL, Najarian JS. Hepatocellular transplantation for metabolic deficiencies: Decrease of plasma bilirubin in Gunn rats. *Science* 1976;192:892–894.
4. Demetriou AA, Whiting JF, Feldman D et al. Replacement of liver function in rats by transplantation of microcarrier-attached hepatocytes. *Science* 1986;233:1190–1192.
5. Margulis MS, Erukhimov EA, Andreiman LA, Viskna LM. Temporary organ substitution by hemoperfusion through suspension of active donor hepatocytes in a total complex of intensive therapy in patients with acute hepatic insufficiency. *Resuscitation* 1989;18:85–94.
6. Rozga J, Holzman MD, Man-soo R et al. Development of a hybrid bioartificial liver. *Ann Surg* 1993;217:502–511.
7. AbouJaoude MM, Grant DR, Ghent CN, Mimeault RE, Wall WJ. Effect of portasystemic shunts on subsequent transplantation of the liver. *Surg Gynecol Obstet* 1991;172:215–219.
8. Rosch JF, Hanafee WN, Snow H. Transjugular portal venography and radiologic portacaval shunt: an experimental study. *Radiology* 1969; 92:1112–1114.
9. Colapinto RF, Stronell RD, Birch SJ, Langer B, Blendis LM, Greig PD, Gilas T. Creation of an intrahepatic portosystemic shunt with a Gruntzig balloon cathter. *Can Med Assoc J* 1982;126:267–268.
10. Laberge JM, Ring EJ, Gordon RL et al. Creation of transjugular intrahepatic portosystemic shunts with the Wallstent endoprostheses: Results in 100 patients. *Radiology* 1993;187:413–420.
11. Ring EJ, Lake JR, Roberts JP et al. Using transjugular intrahepatic portosystemic shunts to control variceal bleeding before liver transplantation. *Ann Intern Med* 1992;116:304–309.
12. Woodle ES, Darcy M, White HM et al. Intrahepatic portosystemic vascular stents: A bridge to hepatic transplantation. *Surgery* 1993;113:344–351.
13. Palmez JC, Garcia F, Sibbitt RR et al. Expandable intrahepatic porta-

caval shunt in dogs with chronic portal hypertension. *Am. J. Radiol* 1986;147:1251–1254.

14. Lind CD, Chong WK, Pinson CW, Richards WO, Mazer M. Transjugular intrahepatic portosystemic shunts (TIPS): Placement for the treatment of portal hypertension and variceal hemorrhage. *Gastroenterology* 1992;102:A843.

21

Implications Concerning the Source of Stem Cells for Bone Marrow Transplantation: Autologous, Allogeneic, Peripheral, and Unrelated

Steven N. Wolff

CASE DESCRIPTION

History

The patient is a 23-year-old female who first presented with back pain in April 1992 which gradually progressed over 1 month to partial paraplegia. A posterior thoracic mass appreciated on physical examination was confirmed by CT scan. Decompressive laminectomy revealed an extradural T2-T8 tumor. Pathologic examination revealed a hematopoietic neoplasm. Karyotypic analysis showed the philadelphia chromosome. DNA southern blotting demonstrated a translocation in the major breakpoint cluster of the BCR gene. Immunoglobulin heavy chain (JH) and immunoglobulin k chain (Jk) gene rearrangement demonstrated clonality. Posterior iliac crest bone marrow exam revealed acute leukemia which was terminal deoxynucleotide (TDT) positive. A diagnosis of lymphoid blastic phase chronic myelogenous leukemia (CML) without an antecedent history of chronic phase disease was made. The patient was treated with chemotherapy consisting of vincristine, prednisone, adriamycin, cyclophosphamide, and intrathecal methotrexate. Complete remission was achieved in June 1992 with resolution of all neurologic manifestations. One month later, repeat bone marrow examination revealed recurrent leukemia and additional chemotherapy was administered. In October 1992, she was referred to Vanderbilt University Medical Center for evaluation and treatment. At that time, the patient was well, without fever, bleeding, weight loss, or weakness but complained of mild night sweats and peripheral neuropathy. Past medical history revealed only routine childhood illnesses. Family and social history demonstrated that the patient was married without children, attending college, and had six siblings, one of which was an identical twin.

Physical Examination

The patient was a pale, alert, and oriented female with normal vital signs. Her gait, HEENT, skin, lymph node, cardiac, pulmonary, and abdominal examinations were normal. Neurologic examination revealed a glove and stocking peripheral neuropathy without other abnormalities.

Laboratory Data

The results of laboratory tests were as follows:

CBC	WBC 2100, PCV 31%, Platelets 182,000, differential 20% neutrophils, 70% lymphocytes, and 10% monocytes.
Electrolytes	Normal
Liver functions	Normal including LDH
Bone marrow	Hypercellular marrow with a proliferation of blasts which were PAS negative, rare sudan black positive, and esterase (specific and non-specific) negative. Immunologic typing revealed CD10, CD19, CD33 and CD34 positivity
EKG	Normal
Chest x-ray	Normal
Spine MRI	Postoperative spinal changes without evidence of mass or signal enhancement
Cardiac mugga	Resting ejection fraction of 53%
PFT	Normal spirometry and DLCO

LP   Normal with no cytologic evidence of leukemia.

HLA typing   See Table 21-1

Hospital Course

Evaluation of the patient revealed residual leukemia in her marrow without evidence of meningeal involvement. Pulmonary, cardiac, renal, and hepatic evaluation revealed normal organ function. A syngeneic marrow transplant was performed on October 15, 1992. The patient received cyclophosphamide (150 mg/kg), VP-16 (1800 mg/m^2), and total body irradiation (1200 cGy) as the preparative marrow transplant regimen. After transplant, low-grade fevers occurred which resolved on broad-spectrum antibiotics. Cyclosporine was administered briefly after transplant to augment autologous (syngeneic) graft-versus-host disease (GVHD). A transient diffuse maculopapular skin rash was noted 2 weeks after transplantation, and skin biopsy was consistent with GVHD. No therapy for GVHD was undertaken and the rash gradually resolved. She was discharged from the hospital on November 9, 1992, 25 days after the transplant. Repeat bone marrow examination did not show leukemia. The patient did well without the need for any medical intervention until April 1, 1993. At that time, 167 days after transplantation, relapse was documented by bone marrow examination. Pres-

Table 21-1.   Histocompatibility Report

Name	Relation	HLA A	HLA B	HLA DR	ABO	Genotype
Annette	Patient	1, 24	44, 62	1, 11	B	AC
Nannette[a]	Sister	1, 24	44, 62	1, 11	B	AC
Donna	Sister	1, 3	7, 44	11, 15	B	AD
Sherry	Sister	1, 3	7, 44	ND[b]	ND	AD
Terry	Sister	1, 3	7, 44	ND	ND	AD
Joseph	Brother	1, 3	7, 44	ND	ND	AD
Robert	Brother	3, X	7, Y	1, 15[c]	ND	BD
Reuben	Father	1, 3	7, 44	11, 15	B	AB
Patricia	Mother	3, 24	7, 62	1, 15	B	CD

[a]Identical twin.

[b]ND not done.

[c]Maternal crossover at DR locus.

Parental genotypic analysis:

   Parent 1 (father): A = A1, B44, DR11
                    B = A3, B7, DR15

   Parent 2 (mother): C = A24, B62, DR1
                    D = A3, B7, DR15

ently, the patient is undergoing additional chemotherapy. A match unrelated donor (MUD) bone marrow transplant (BMT) is being contemplated.

CASE DISCUSSION

Our patient had refractory acute biphenotypic leukemia which was unlikely to respond to additional standard chemotherapy. Bone marrow transplantation (BMT) was judged to offer her the best likelihood of long-term leukemia control. In determining which type of BMT is most feasible, complete HLA evaluation of the extended family was performed (Table 21-1). This evaluation revealed no suitable donors other than the identical twin.

Chronic myelogenous leukemia usually presents as myeloid proliferation with myeloid maturation termed the chronic phase. The hematologic picture is an elevated white blood count, a left shifted differential with increased eosinophils, and basophils. Thrombocytosis can occur and infrequently may be the sole hematologic manifestation. The philadelphia chromosome is detected in over 90% of cases and represents a translocation between chromosomes 9 and 22. The Abelson proto-oncogene on chromosome 9 is transferred to the BCR gene on chromosome 22 in a region called the major breakpoint cluster. Using DNA southern blotting or RNA pcr technology, this translocation is detected in over 99% of all CML patients [1]. The protein product (p210) of this translocated gene is a highly active tyrosine kinase that contributes to cellular proliferation. CML is an inexorable progressive disease with acute leukemia (blastic phase) being the terminal event. The median duration of the chronic phase prior to blast crisis is 3.5 years. Some patients have no detectable chronic phase and are first detected in blast phase. Blastic phase CML can be myeloid, lymphoid (commonly B cell), or biphenotypic. Up to 25% of adult acute lymphocytic leukemia (ALL) can be philadelphia chromosome positive. The translocation in this leukemia occurs outside of the major breakpoint cluster designated as the minor breakpoint cluster region. The location of the translocation is helpful in determining whether de novo ALL is lymphoid blastic phase CML. Philadelphia chromosome positive de novo acute myeloid leukemia is blastic phase CML.

The chemotherapy treatment of blastic phase CML is disappointing. Myeloid blastic phase CML is generally refractory to chemotherapy. Most patients survive only 1–3 months. Recent investigations have revealed a high content of cell membrane p-glycoprotein (pgp), suggesting one biochemical mechanism for profound chemotherapy resistance. Lymphoid blastic phase CML can respond to standard ALL therapy (vincristine and prednisone) but generally relapses and resists further therapy. There is a substantial incidence of central nervous system disease (meningeal) and extramedullary disease (chloroma) with blastic phase CML.

Compared to standard therapy, BMT offers some curative potential for blastic phase CML [2–4]. Substantially improved survival is, however, achieved if patients are transplanted prior to blast crisis. BMT administers supraintensive chemotherapy and radiation therapy (preparative regimen). This substantial increment in dose can eradicate leukemias that are incurable with less intensive therapy. Substantial damage to the residual normal hematopoietic stem cells result from the intensive therapy. After supraintensive therapy, the bone marrow transplant is required to regenerate hematopoiesis. Patients would have severe and unrelenting bone marrow hypoplasia (aplastic anemia) without the bone marrow reinfusion (transplant).

The source of stem cells is an important determinant of the success of the marrow transplant (Table 21-2). Readily available sources include the patient's own marrow (autologous or AUTO), the patient's peripheral blood (peripheral stem cell or PBSC), a matched family member (related allogeneic or ALLO), an identical twin (syngeneic), or a matched unrelated donor (MUD). Other sources such as fetal liver or umbilical cord blood are novel investigative approaches not readily available.

Autologous bone marrow transplants (ABMT) and PBSC transplants are used for patients whose primary disease does not reside in the marrow or whose marrows have been cleared of recognizable abnormal elements by prior chemotherapy [5–6]. This transplant is readily available, because an HLA-matched donor is not required.

Autologous bone marrow stem cells are collected by multiple posterior iliac crest aspirations while the patient is under general or regional anesthesia. The collected marrow is red blood cell depleted and cryopreserved for later use. PBSC are collected by multiple peripheral

Table 21-2. Relative Comparison of Sources of Hematopoietic Stem Cells

Source	Availability	Graft Failure	Tumor Content	GVHD	GVL	Relapse
AUTO	+++	+/−	+++	+/−	+/−	++++
PBSC	++++	+/−	++	+/−	+/−	+++
ALLO	+	+	−	+++	+++	++
MUD	++	++	−	++++	++++	+

blood leukapheresis procedures without the necessity of anesthesia. PBSC collections require stem cell mobilization from the marrow to the peripheral blood. Mobilization can be accomplished by growth factors that greatly increase the number of marrow stem cells migrating to the peripheral blood. Augmented numbers of peripheral stem cells also occur after recovery from routine chemotherapy. A common method for mobilizing PBSC is chemotherapy followed by hematopoietic growth factors (dual mobilization). The leukapheresis is performed when mobilized stem cells are first detected by either a rising white blood cell count or assaying for CD34 positive blood mononuclear cells. After chemotherapy, CD34 positive cells appear prior to normalization of peripheral blood counts. PBSC are cryopreserved similarly to autologous bone marrow.

For transplantation, the cryopreserved stem cells are thawed, infused intravenously, migrate to the marrow, and slowly mature and regenerate. Adequate hematopoiesis is achieved 2–4 weeks after transplantation and is fostered by the use of growth factors such as gm-csf and g-csf. Patients whose marrows are heavily pretreated with chemotherapy or radiation prior to harvest are more likely to have inadequate recovery of hematopoiesis. PBSC transplants may more rapidly recover white blood cell and platelet counts than other forms of transplantation. AUTO BMT or PBSC transplants are less morbid compared to ALLO BMT with fewer infectious complications. The reinfusion of occult leukemia residing in the marrow or peripheral blood is a risk, as the transplant is performed after completion of all cytotoxic therapy. The marrow or peripheral blood can be ex vivo purged using chemotherapy or immunologic methods if occult leukemia contamination is possible. Without immunologic differences between patient and donor, graft failure is uncommon.

The major limitation of ABMT or PBSC transplants is relapse. There is less experience using PBSC transplants, but recent information has suggested that relapse may be reduced compared to AUTO BMT. Because the donor and the patient are the same, it is difficult to assess whether relapse is due to the incomplete eradication of the leukemia remaining in the patient and/or contamination of the harvested stem cells with occult leukemia. Retroviral vector labeling of cells may provide a clue to the source of relapse after transplantation.

ALLO BMT is performed after HLA evaluation of donor and recipient. Unlike solid organ transplants, ALLO BMT or MUD BMT require complete or near HLA identity. The histocompatibility requirement is a six or five antigen match at all HLA, A, B, and DR loci. Allogeneic marrow is collected from the normal donor the day of the transplant using techniques similar to AUTO BMT harvests. If red blood cell or plasma incompatibility exist, the marrow is ex vivo red blood cell or plasma depleted prior to reinfusion.

Allogeneic transplants differ from other transplants because of graft-versus-host disease (GVHD). Although HLA compatible, allogeneic transplants still have some major and minor HLA differences. Marrow transplants regenerate immune competent donor cells that can recognize and react against host tissues. GVHD can lead to organ failure, impaired hematopoiesis, decreased overall immunocompetence, and various infections. The incidence and severity of GVHD increase with HLA disparity. More than one antigen disparate transplants are not routinely performed. Due to GVHD, allogeneic transplants are more morbid than autologous transplants. In many diseases, survival is not reduced because of a substantially diminished risk of relapse. The reduced risk of relapse is due to immunologic destruction of remaining leukemia by the immunologic competent donor cells. This process is termed graft-versus-leukemia (GVL). Theoretically, GVHD and GVL do not occur after autologous bone marrow transplants. However, in rare cases, autoreactivity can be described after AUTO BMT and may be initiated by brief use of cyclosporine. PBSC transplants have a much higher content of T lymphocytes compared to AUTO BMT. These cells may contribute to autologous GVHD, which may be the reason why relapse is less frequent after PBSC transplants compared to AUTO BMT. The other advantage of allogeneic transplants is the elimination of the possibility of leukemia contamination of the transplanted marrow, as the stem cells are provided by a normal healthy donor.

MUD marrow transplants are now feasible with the success of donor programs, most notably the National Marrow Donor Program (NMDP). The NMDP has over 700,000 HLA-typed volunteers. Volunteer marrow donors are possible, as harvesting of marrow is not dangerous and does not result in donor marrow dysfunction. This large donor pool is required, considering the genetic polymorphism of the human HLA system and the requirement for complete donor HLA identity. This type of transplant is reserved for the patient who requires an allogeneic source of marrow but has no compatible family donor. The patient and donor need to be scrutinously matched because GVHD is highly prevalent after MUD BMT. Presently, the NMDP is matching class II antigens (HLA DR) by site-specific oligonucleotide DNA probes. Concomitant with increased GVHD, GVL is very likely and relapse is lowest for this type of transplant. Presently, the high morbidity of MUD GVHD negates the survival advantage of MUD GVL.

Syngeneic marrow transplant represents an infrequent opportunity to evaluate the various parameters leading to the success of transplantation. In this type of marrow transplant, a genotypically identical individual serves as the source of marrow. Thus, GVHD and GVL are eliminated along with the possibility of leukemia marrow contamination. This form of transplant is the least morbid and has an intermediary risk of relapse compared to other transplants. Without GVL, syngeneic marrow transplants have a higher risk of relapse compared to ALLO BMT. Without tumor cell contamination, syngeneic marrow transplants have a lower risk of relapse compared to AUTO BMT.

The decision of which type of marrow to use as the source of stem cells is based on donor availability, the physiologic state of the patient, the risk of occult patient marrow leukemia contamination, the age of the patient, and the risk of relapse. In circumstances where the risk of relapse after transplantation is substantial, an allogeneic source of marrow may be preferred.

The realm of BMT is rapidly changing. Improved methods to eliminate occult leukemia contamination of the marrow are available. Improved methods to prevent and treat GVHD are under investigation. Experimental models of eliciting GVL without GVHD are under development. Considering this changing environment, the choice of which type of marrow transplant to pursue is sometimes difficult and is the subject of comparative clinical research studies.

REFERENCES

1. Epner DE, Koeffler HP. Molecular genetic advances in chronic myelogenous leukemia. *Ann Intern Med* 1990;113:3–6.
2. Champlin R. Bone marrow transplantation for chronic myelogenous leukemia. *Curr Opin Oncol* 1990;2(2):258–262.
3. Snyder DS, McGlave PB. Treatment of chronic myelogenous leukemia with bone marrow transplantation. *Hematol Oncol Clin North Amer* 1990;4(3):535–557.
4. Liner CA. Treatment of acute leukemia in adults. *Curr Opin Oncol* 1992;4(1):53–65.
5. Inwards D, Kessinger A. Peripheral blood stem cell transplantation: Historical prospective, current status and prospects for the future. *Transfus Med Rev* 1992;6(3):183–190.
6. Hess AD, Jones RJ, Morris LE, Noga SJ, Yeager AM, Vogelsang GB, Santos GW. Autologous graft-versus-host disease: A new frontier in immunotherapy. *Bone Marrow Transplant* 1992;10 (Suppl. 1):16–21.

22

Graft-Versus-Host Disease

J. Greer

The patient is a 22-year-old white female who was diagnosed with acute myelocytic leukemia when she was noted to have leucocytosis after a motor vehicle accident. She went into remission with "7 and 3" (cytosine arabinoside and daunomycin) and was consolidated with high-dose cytosine arabinoside (3 g/m^2 q 12h × 12, days 1–6) and daunomycin (30 mg/m^2 × 3 days, days 7–9) in March 1988. She did well until 21 months after remission when blasts were noted in her peripheral blood; WBC = 14.0 × 10 cells/mm^3 (differential: 2% neutrophils, 2% metamyelocytes, 48% blasts, 28% lymphocytes, 20% monocytes), platelet = 30 × 10 cell/mm^3, and hematocrit = 30%.

She subsequently underwent an allogeneic bone marrow transplant from her HLA-matched sister. The patient was cytomegalovirus (CMV) seropositive. The preparative regimen was etoposide (1800 mg/m^2 over 26 h), cyclophosphamide (50 mg/kg/day × 3 days) with mesna, and total body irradiation (1000 rads over 3 days). Her graft-versus-host disease (GVHD) prophylaxis was cyclosporine (1.5 mg/kg q 12h) and short course methotrexate (15 mg/m^2 on day 1, 10 mg/m^2 on days 3, 6, and 11); however, she did not receive day 11 methotrexate due to severe mucositis. She received broad-spectrum antibiotics early due to fever on day −3 and she also received prophylactic acyclovir and fluconazole. Amphotericin B was substituted for fluconazole on day 9 due to persistent fever and mucositis. On day 11, blood cultures became positive for coagulase positive staphylococcus; vancomycin was added to the antibiotics. Engraftment started on day 15 when WBC was 1.3 × 10^3 with 68% neutrophils; platelets remained over 30 × 10^3 after day 17. She developed infiltrates on day 17, but bronchoscopy was negative on day 18. The patient continued to have nausea and vomiting; the intravenous antibiotics were discontinued on day 28.

Diarrhea occurred on day 29 and a maculopapular rash was noted on her forearms and palms on day 32; bilirubin was 0.7 mg/dl. Skin biopsy was positive for GVHD and the patient was started on steroids (prednisone at 1 mg/kg q 12h) on day 34. She became febrile on day 37, had intermittent abdominal pain, and an episode of hypotension on day 38. Broad-spectrum antibiotics were restarted on day 37; bilirubin was increased at 2.6 mg/dl and albumin dropped to 1.9 mg/dl. Steroids were increased (medrol at 2 mg/kg q 12h) on day 42 because of worsening GVHD (rash, diarrhea, bilirubin = 4.1 mg/dl). She gradually improved and was able to be discharged on day 55; discharge medications included medrol, cyclosporine, trimethoprim/sufamethoxazole, and weekly intravenous gamma-globulin. She required a brief hospitalization on days 137–142 due to diarrhea which was secondary to *Clostridium difficile* infection. Her skin has gradually improved, but she has had recurrent bronchitis, an episode of shingles, and a mild sicca syndrome. She is presently doing well over $3\frac{1}{2}$ years from her transplant, with limited skin chronic GVHD, normal liver functions, and no evidence of leukemia.

Allogeneic bone marrow transplantation in animals identified a "secondary" or "runting" syndrome within 20–30 days of transplantation that was characterized by weight loss, diarrhea, skin lesions, and necrosis of liver cells. In 1966, Billingham established the criteria for the development of GVHD: (1) the graft must contain immunologically competent cells; (2) the host must contain antigens that are lacking in the graft and will stimulate the graft to respond to the antigens; and (3) the host is unable to mount an effective immunological reaction against the graft which has developed "security of tenure." Subsequent investigations have identified GVHD as a T-cell-mediated process. GVHD is subdivided into acute (before 100 days) and chronic (after 100 days), although the separation is often indistinct in the cyclosporine era [1–5].

The target organs of *acute GVHD* are skin, liver, and gastrointestinal tract, and the severity of GVHD can be given an overall grade using clinical and pathological criteria (Table 22-1). The most serious aspect of acute GVHD is gastrointestinal involvement which may result in ileus,

Table 22-1. Acute GVHD

(a) Staging by Organ System			(b) Overall Clinical Grade					
Organ	Extent of Involvement	Stage	I	II$_{SLI}$	II$_S$	II$_{LI}$	III	IV
Skin (S)	Rash (% of body surface) <25	+						
	25–50	++						
	>50	+++						
	Bullae, desquamation	++++						
Liver (L)	Bilirubin (mg%) 2–3	+						
	3.1–6	++						
	6.1–15	+++						
	>15	++++						
Intestine (I)	Diarrhea (ml/day) >500	+						
	>1000	++						
	>1500	+++						
	Pain/Ileus	++++						

Source: Adapted from Deeg HJ and Cottler-Fox M. Clinical spectrum and pathophysiology of acute graft-vs-host disease. In: Barakoff SJ et al. eds. *Graft-vs-Host Disease Immunology, Pathophysiology, and Treatment*. New York: Marcel Dekker, Inc., 1990.

perforation, and peritonitis. The incidence of GVHD is variable with rates of 20–70%, and risk factors for its development include patient (and donor) age, sex mismatch between donor and patient (in particular, transplants from allosensitized females into male recipients), histoincompatibility, and the presence of certain HLA-A or -B alleles.

Prophylaxis of GVHD has primarily involved drug therapy but can also involve the depletion of donor T cells from the marrow graft by a variety of methods including monoclonal antibodies, soybean lectin, and elutriation. Several centers have performed randomized trials indicating that two drugs are better than one in decreasing GVHD. The University of Minnesota reported a 48% incidence of GVHD in patients receiving methotrexate alone compared to 21% in patients who received methotrexate, antithymocyte globulin, and prednisone (p = .001). Investigators at the Fred Hutchinson Cancer Research Center reported a 54% incidence of GVHD in patients receiving cyclosporine alone compared to 33% with cyclosporine and methotrexate (p = .014); they subsequently found no benefit to adding prednisone to the combination regimen. New immunosuppressive agents, such as FK-506, may improve GVHD prophylaxis. T-depletion of the donor marrow does decrease GVHD; however, there may be decreased engraftment, increased relapse, and the development of lymphoproliferative disorders. Further work on selective T-depletion is required to try to optimize the decreased GVHD without the introduction of new problems.

The development of acute GVHD, by definition, indicates prophylaxis failed; and therapy depends, in part, on the drugs used for prophylaxis. In general, corticosteroid therapy in high doses is usually the initial therapy for acute GVHD. Response rates vary from 30% to 70%, but mortality due to opportunistic infections and interstitial pneumonitis is high. Antithymocyte globulin (ATG) may be added to therapy of acute GVHD with similar response rates; cytopenias, fever, chills, allergic reactions, and serum sickness may occur with ATG therapy. Monoclonal antibody therapy usually directed at T cells has primarily been used in steroid-resistant patients, and response rates over 50% have been reported; however, mortality remains high due to infections and recurrence of GVHD. More specific monoclonal antibody therapy given earlier in the course of acute GVHD may eventually prove beneficial.

Chronic GVHD has more autoimmune features than acute GVHD and can occur in three settings: (1) progressive onset as an extension of acute GVHD; (2) quiescent onset after an interval in which acute GVHD is controlled; (3) de novo presentation without any preceding acute GVHD. Any acute GVHD increases the risk of chronic GVHD, and a progressive onset is associated with a worse prognosis. Chronic GVHD can be subdivided into limited and extensive stage according to the severity of skin and liver involvement (Table 22-2).

Chronic GVHD often produces a sicca syndrome and, over time, may resemble scleroderma with induration and atrophy of skin and joint contractures. Liver involvement is usually characterized by cholestasis but rarely progresses to cirrhosis. Severe mucositis of the mouth and esophagus can result in weight loss, but lower gastrointestinal tract involvement is unusual. The lungs are usually not considered target organs for GVHD but may have abnormalities varying from steroid-sensitive lymphocytic interstitial infiltrates to progressive bronchiolitis obliterans. The hematopoietic system may be affected with eosinophilia and persistent thrombocytopenia, the latter being associated with a poor outcome in chronic GVHD. Rarely, polymyositis, neuropathy, and nephrotic syndrome have been attributed to chronic GVHD.

A major problem of GVHD is the increased risk of opportunistic infections. Cytomegalovirus, fungal infections, bacteremias, viral infections, bacteremias, viral infections, and *pneumocystis carinii* may all occur due to immunosuppressive therapy but also to delayed immune recovery secondary to GVHD. Specific abnormalities in immunity include low gamma-globulin levels, functional asplenia, impaired antibody responses to specific antigens, and decreases in the number and function of CD4+ T cells. Immunological recovery usually occurs within 1–2 years of an uncomplicated allogeneic marrow transplant but is significantly delayed with chronic GVHD. Prophylactic antibiotics and anti-

Table 22-2. Chronic GVHD

Type	Extent of Disease
Limited	Localized skin involvement and/or liver dysfunction
Extensive	Generalized skin involvement
	Localized skin involvement or liver dysfunction with one of the following:

- Chronic agressive hepatitis, bridging necrosis, or cirrhosis
- Sicca syndrome
    Eye involvement (Schirmer's <5 mm)
    Mucosalivary gland involvement
    Mucosal involvement (on lip biopsy)
- Involvement of other organs

Source: Adapted from Shulman HM, Sullivan KM, Weiden PL et al. Chronic graft versus host syndrome in man: A long-term clinicopathologic study of 20 Seattle patients. *Am J Med* 69;204:1980.

viral agents are warranted in all patients to decrease infections. Additionally, intravenous gamma-globulin ameliorates the course of GVHD.

Therapy of chronic GVHD is controversial but usually includes one or more immunosuppressive agents [2–5]. Because long-term administration of cyclosporine may be associated with a decreased risk of chronic GVHD, a slow taper of cyclosporine may be warranted in allogeneic transplantation, at a rate of 5% per week starting around day 50 and completing around day 180. Acute flares of GVHD may occur during the taper and require reinstitution of immunosuppressive therapy. Alternate-day steroids and cyclosporine have had response rates over 50% in patients with chronic GVHD at the Fred Hutchinson Cancer Research Center. Investigators at Johns Hopkins have indicated a role for thalidomide in the treatment of refractory chronic GVHD. There may also be a role for PUVA (psoralen with ultraviolet light) therapy or extracorporeal photophoresis for patients with significant chronic GVHD involving the skin, and ursodeoxycholic acid for liver involvement. New strategies in the treatment of GVHD may involve the introduction of cytokines. Preliminary animal and human data indicate less GVHD in patients receiving GM-CSF after allogeneic marrow transplantation. A hypothesis of the benefit of GM-CSF is that early neutrophil recovery is associated with healing of gastrointestinal ulcerations and less exposure to bacterial antigens that can promote GVHD.

Whereas decreasing the severity of GVHD is an important goal in marrow transplantation, maintaining the *graft versus leukemia* (GVL) *effect* to decrease relapse rates is equally as important. Weiden and colleagues in Seattle recognized in the 1970s the decreased relapse rates in patients experiencing GVHD compared to patients who had either no GVHD or had undergone syngeneic marrow transplants. The GVL effect has been most pronounced in those patients who are considered at high risk for relapse, that is, patients with chronic granulocytic leukemia in accelerated or blast crisis and relapsed acute leukemias.

In this case report, the patient had severe acute GVHD manifested by diffuse skin changes and gastrointestinal involvement with probable peritonitis and sepsis. The disease was controlled with high-dose steroids. She subsequently developed chronic GVHD manifested by a sicca syndrome, recurrent bacterial infections, and low gamma-globulin levels. She was maintained on prophylactic antibiotics and gamma-globulin and is doing well over 3 years out from transplantation. She is considered high risk because she was transplanted in relapse; however, she has not relapsed, in part due to the graft versus leukemia effect.

REFERENCES

1. Vogelsang GB, Hess AD, Santos GW. Acute graft-versus-host disease: Clinical characteristics in the cyclosporine era. *Medicine* 1988;67:163–174.
2. Deeg HJ, Henslee-Downey PJ. Management of acute graft-versus-host disease. *Bone Marrow Transplant* 1990;6:1–8.
3. Sullivan KM, Weiden PL, Storb R et al. Influence of acute and chronic graft-versus-host disease on relapse and survival after bone marrow transplantation from HL-identical siblings as treatment of acute and chronic leukemia. *Blood* 1989;73:1720–1728.
4. Wingard JR, Piantadosi S, Vogelsang GB, Farmer ER, Jabs DA, Levin LS, Bescharner WE, Cahill RA, Miller DF, Harrison D, Saral R, Santos GW. Predictors of death from chronic graft-versus host disease after bone marrow transplantation. *Blood* 1989;74:1428–1435.
5. Ferrara JLM, Deeg HJ. Graft-versus-host disease. *N Engl J Med* 1991;324:667–674.

23

Veno-occlusive Disease of the Liver in Bone Marrow Transplantation

Richard S. Stein

SC, a 31-year-old woman, presented to her physician in June 1992 having experienced fever, night sweats, and weight loss, and having noted left upper quadrant fullness. Workup revealed splenomegaly, but the physical examination was otherwise unremarkable. Blood counts included hematocrit 34%, platelets 788,000/mm^3, and white blood cell count 317,000/mm^3. The differential was 21 neutrophils, 24 bands, 19 metamyelocytes, 26 myelocytes, 6 promyelocytes, and 4 blasts. Bone marrow aspirate and biopsy revealed a hypercellular marrow with myeloid hyperplasia; bone marrow karyotype analysis revealed the presence of a 9;22 translocation, that is, the philadelphia chromosome, with many cells showing a second philadelphia chromosome. The diagnosis of chronic granulocytic leukemia was made. There was no past history of liver disease, and serologic studies revealed no evidence of past or present infection with hepatitis A, B, or C, or by cytomegalovirus. She was started on hydrea to control her counts and was referred to Vanderbilt University Medical Center for evaluation for bone marrow transplantation.

The patient's brother was identified as an appropriate allogeneic donor as he was identical at five of six HLA A,B,DR loci. Because of the double philadelphia chromosome, the patient was felt to be at risk for an accelerated clinical course and was, therefore, admitted on October 20, 1992 for placement of a Hickman catheter and allogeneic bone marrow transplantation. The preparative regimen included VP-16, 1800 mg/m^2 on day -7, cyclophosphamide 50 mg/kg/day on days -6, -5, and -4, and total body irradiation, twice a day for six fractions, 200 rads per fraction, on days -3, -2, and -1. For prophylaxis against graft-versus-host disease the patient received cyclosporine 1.5 mg/kg I.V. over 2 h every 12 h, starting on day -1; methotrexate was administered at a dose of 10 mg/m^2 on days 1, 3, and 6. As antibiotic prophylaxis, the patient received vancomycin 1 g I.V. q 12h, starting day -1, ciprofloxacin 500 mg P.O. q 12h, starting day -1, acyclovir 400 mg I.V. q 12h, starting day -1, and fluconazole 400 mg P.O. qd starting day -1.

On October 30, 1992 the patient received bone marrow from her brother. The posttransplant course was complicated by fever, which responded to continued antibiotics and to the institution of amphotericin B. The patient also experienced vaginal bleeding, which was treated with premarin and provera but which persisted for several weeks. Oral mucositis necessitated the use of dilaudid.

The serum bilirubin was noted to be elevated (2.9 mg/dl) on day 6 (Table 23-1). Over the next 18 days, the bilirubin rose to a peak level of 27.2 mg/dl; during this time an increase in weight (114 to 121 pounds) and abdominal girth (24 to 28 in.) were also noted. The serum alkaline

Table 23-1. Lab Data of Index Patient After BMT

Date	Day	Bilirubin (mg/dl)	SGOT (IU/dl)	Weight	Creatinine (mg/dl)
10/20	−10	0.4	13	114	0.5
10/29	−1	0.4	24	114	0.3
11/04	5	0.9	17	115	0.4
11/05	6	2.9	12	115	0.3
11/09	10	5.6	13	110	0.3
11/11	12	7.4	11	114	0.7
11/12	13	10.5	9	116	0.6
11/13	14	12.5	8	115	0.8
11/16	17	12.1	8	121	1.3
11/18	19	15.8	8	123	1.1
11/19	20	20.2	4	119	1.1
11/23	24	27.2	9	116	1.4
11/25	26	24.8	9	115	1.0
11/26	27	21.6	11	115	1.0
11/29	30	16.9	14	117	0.9
12/02	33	13.1	23	114	1.1
12/03	34	14.3	24	111	1.1
12/07	38	11.8	32	104	1.2
12/11	41	4.5	40	103	1.3

phosphatase and asportate aminotransferase (SGOT) remained normal despite the rise in bilirubin. In the absence of an alternative etiology, the diagnosis of veno-occlusive disease (VOD) of the liver was made.

Treatment of VOD consisted of careful management of her intravascular volume status, including infusions of albumin. The cyclosporin dose was adjusted to maintain therapeutic levels. The use of heparin and/or tissue plasminogen activator (TPA) was considered. However, because of persistent vaginal bleeding, therapy was essentially limited to supportive care and pentoxyfilline 400 mg P.O. tid starting on day 15. The bilirubin gradually returned to the normal range.

Bone marrow engraftment occurred as shown by a WBC of 3.9 with 88% granulocytes on day 24; there was no evidence of graft-versus-host disease during this hospitalization. The patient was discharged on day 43 following transplant, at which time the bilirubin was 4.5 mg/dl. The bilirubin normalized after discharge.

DISCUSSION

Long-term survival following bone marrow transplantation (BMT) for malignancy requires elimination of the malignancy, engraftment by the donor bone marrow, and successful management of both graft-versus-host disease, and of the other complications that can occur following BMT and that represent either regimen-related toxicity or complications secondary to transplant-related immunosuppression.

A critical complication of bone marrow transplantation which is illustrated by this patient is the syndrome of liver damage covered by the term veno-occlusive disease (VOD). VOD involves fibrous obliteration of small hepatic venules and small sublobular veins, and the histopathology also involves pericentral hepatocyte necrosis and congestion. VOD is the third leading cause of death following BMT, exceeded by graft-versus-host disease in patients undergoing allogeneic BMT and exceeded only by infection in patients undergoing autologous BMT. Although the syndrome of VOD is associated with a histopathologic description, in reality, liver biopsies are rarely performed in the immediate posttransplant period, and VOD is diagnosed on clinical rather than pathologic grounds.

VOD is diagnosed when two of the three following events occur within 20 days of bone marrow transplantation in the absence of another explanation of the signs and symptoms: hyperbilirubinemia >2 mg/dl, hepatomegaly or right upper quadrant pain of liver origin, and sudden weight gain >2% of baseline body weight because of fluid accumulation.

From the earliest publications on VOD it has been clear that the risk of VOD is greater in patients receiving high-dose cytoreductive therapy than in patients receiving low-dose cytoreductive therapy. Over the past decade, therapeutic regimens used in conjunction with BMT have become more dose intense, and the patients receiving BMT have often received more intense primary therapy for their malignant diseases. It is, therefore, not surprising that a recent study noted that over the past decade the incidence of VOD had risen. What is surprising is the magnitude of the increase. Using the same diagnostic criteria, the authors reported that the incidence of VOD had increased from 21% in 1980 to 54% in 1987–1988 and that 15% of patients developed severe VOD; severe VOD was associated with death in all but one patient.

In addition to the intensity of cytoreductive therapy, a number of risk factors for the development of VOD have been identified. These factors include elevated pretransplant aspartate aminotransferase (SGOT) levels, administration of acyclovir or vancomycin, administration of mismatched or unrelated donor bone marrow, and previous radiotherapy to the abdomen. It should be noted that it is not clear if an apparent risk factor is directly related to VOD or if the factor serves as a marker of other processes that predispose to VOD. Specifically, vancomycin and acyclovir may be markers for infectious processes that increase the risk of VOD. Similarly, the use of T-cell-depleted donor bone marrow has been associated with a decreased risk of VOD; this may well be due to the fact that T-cell-depletion eliminates the need for administration of methotrexate and cyclosporin as prophylaxis for GVHD, and such therapy has been identified as a risk factor in other studies.

If VOD is due to the intensity of therapy and the occurrence of coexistent problems causing liver damage, there would appear to be no obvious way to decrease VOD without producing a trade-off in increased deaths due to tumor relapse or due to the exclusion of patients from therapy protocols. In this context, it would, therefore, be reassuring if effective therapy of VOD existed. Unfortunately, the basic therapy of VOD is supportive. To prevent additional complications such as renal failure, intravascular volume should be maintained by transfusions of red cells and colloid, and electrolytes should be closely monitored. Other therapy of VOD is experimental. Based on the histopathologic appearance of VOD, low-dose heparin has been advocated as a means of preventing VOD. The results of such trials have not been consistently favorable, and due to the complex etiology of VOD, it might well be that heparin schedules effective in the context of some preparative regimens might be ineffective in others. Recombinant tissue plasminogen activator (TPA) has been used to treat VOD in a limited population, and whereas the safety of the drug has been shown, the efficacy of the treatment and the applicability to the wide range of patients with VOD has not been established. Pentoxifylline has been advocated as a means of blocking TNF-alpha, but the effectiveness of such therapy has not yet been proven.

In summary, as preparative regimens used in conjunction with bone marrow transplant have become more aggressive, VOD has become a more common clinical problem. At present, the standard therapy is to provide supportive care in the hopes that the disorder will run its course and reverse as in our present patient. Successful treatment of VOD clearly is becoming one of the major challenges for bone marrow transplantation in this decade.

BIBLIOGRAPHY

ATTAL M, HUGUET F, RUBIE H et al. Prevention of hepatic veno-occlusive disease after bone marrow transplantation by continuous infusion of low dose heparin: A prospective, randomized trial. *Blood* 1992;79:2834–2840.

ESSELL JH, THOMPSON JM, HARMAN GS et al. Marked Increase in veno-occlusive disease of the liver associated with methotrexate use for graft-versus-host disease prophylaxis in patients receiving busulfan/cyclophosphamide. *Blood* 1992;79:2784–2788.

MCDONALD GB, SHARMA P, MATTHEWS DE et al. The clinical course of 53 patients with venocclusive disease of the liver after marrow transplantation. *Transplantation* 1985;39:603–607.

MCDONALD GB, HINDS MS, FISHER LD et al. Veno-occlusive disease of the liver and multiorgan failure after bone marrow transplantation: A cohort of 355 patients. *Ann Intern Med* 1993;118:255–267.

SHULMAN HM, HINTERBERGER W. Hepatic veno-occlusive disease—Liver toxicity syndrome after bone marrow transplantation. *Bone Marrow Transplant* 1992;10:197–214.

24

A Bone Marrow Transplant Recipient with Fever and Hematuria

Stephen Dummer and Joseph Horvath

A 22-year-old black man presented to an outside physician complaining of bleeding gums and fatigue. Studies of peripheral blood and bone marrow were consistent with aplastic anemia. There was no history of viral hepatitis or exposure to drugs or chemicals toxic to the bone marrow. He received an allogeneic bone marrow transplant from his sister, matched at five out of six HLA loci. Pretransplant conditioning included total lymphoid irradiation and cyclophosphamide. Graft-versus-host prophylaxis included cyclosporine, methotrexate, and weekly intravenous immunoglobulin. His posttransplant course was complicated by *Enterobacter cloacae* bacteremia and acute graft-versus-host disease, but he recovered and was discharged 42 days after transplantation.

On day 67 after transplantation he was seen in clinic and was doing well. His white blood cell count was 5,700 his hematocrit 36.0, and platelet count 55,000. He was maintained on 40 mg bid of methylprednisolone for graft-versus-host disease. Later that evening he developed acute left flank pain, hematuria, and loose stools. He denied fever, chills, nausea, vomiting, cough, headache, or shortness of breath. He was admitted to an outside hospital the next day and was found to have hydronephrosis on the right side. A cystoscopy showed blood clots obstructing the distal ureter but no hemorrhagic cystitis. A stent was placed. On the third hospital day he developed a fever of 104°F. The urine specimen from admission was growing adenovirus in tissue culture. He was transferred to Vanderbilt University. Upon arrival, he was on methylprednisolone 40 mg twice a day, cyclosporine 260 mg twice a day, fluconazole, vancomycin, and imipenem. He had also been receiving daily prophylaxis with sulfmethoxazole–trimethoprim, but this had been discontinued 8 days earlier. The physical exam showed a healthy black male in mild distress from flank pain. He was afebrile with a pulse of 80, respiration rate of 20, and blood pressure of 130/80. His exam was remarkable for a few petechiae over his soft palate. No lymphadenopathy was noted. His lungs were clear, and the heart rhythm was regular with no murmurs or rubs. His abdomen was remarkable for the absence of hepatosplenomegaly. There was tenderness in the right lower quadrant. He also had tenderness in the right flank area. The extremities were remarkable only for skin changes consistent with mild graft-versus-host disease.

LABORATORY EXAM

Laboratory studies showed a white blood cell count of 2000, a hematocrit of 29.0, and a platelet count of 26,000. The differential was 94 polys, 4 monocytes, 2 lymphocytes, and 4 nucleated red cells. BUN and creatinine were 29 mg/dl and 1.7 mg/dl, respectively. Other chemistries were remarkable for a creatinine phosphkinase of 466, an alkaline phosphatase of 60, and an SGOT of 48. The bilirubin was normal. Urinalysis showed numerous red blood cells and five to six white blood cells per high-power field. A room air blood gas showed a pH of 7.48, pCO_2 of 32, and pO_2 of 52. A Ventilation/perfusion scan was performed and interpreted as showing a low probability for pulmonary embolus.

HOSPITAL COURSE

The patient was placed on clindamycin and ciprofloxacin. Later that evening he had a fever to 105°F. By the second hospital day, the admission urine culture was growing adenovirus, subsequently found to be type 11. A quantitative culture showed 10^7 infectious particles per milliliter of urine. The patients hypoxemia improved slightly and his chest radiograph was clear. On the third hospital day, he developed abdominal pain and distention. A CT scan of the abdomen showed a thickening of the cecal wall but no definite abscess or perforation. Stool studies were negative for *Clostridium difficile* and bacterial pathogens.

The fever, hypoxemia, hydronephrosis, and hematuria were all thought to be a result of disseminated adenovirus infection. Based on in vitro data that some strains of adenovirus were susceptible to achievable serum levels of ganciclovir, he was begun on ganciclovir 5 mg/kg every 8 h. Three days into this treatment, his temperature was still 105°F, and his white count had dropped to 600. Pulmonary function tests showed moderate restrictive disease but a normal diffusing capacity. Three days later, his white count had increased to 2000; however, he remained febrile to 103.6°F, and now developed an acute hydronephrosis on the left with subsequent decreased urine output. Bilateral ureteral stents were placed, but his renal function did not improve. The patient then developed increasing abdominal pain and abdominal distention requiring placement of a nasogastric tube. This, however, led to pharyngeal hemorrhage and necessitated intubation. On the next day, bilateral nephrostomy tubes were placed, but urine flow remained minimal due to persistence of blood clots obstructing the nephrostomy tubes. Adenovirus was repeatedly isolated from his urine. Complement fixation titers for adenovirus rose from 1 : 8 on admission to 1 : 64 on hospital day 16. On hospital day 11, hemodialysis was begun because of anuria. Daily fevers as high as 105°F persisted. His white blood cell count dropped below 1000, and on hospital day 12, the ganciclovir was discontinued. Blood cultures remained negative for other viruses, bacteria or fungi. On hospital day 19, he developed progressive hypoxemia, refractory hypotension, bradycardia, and subsequently expired. Postmortem exam was refused.

DISCUSSION

Adenoviruses are a closely related group of double-stranded, nonenveloped DNA viruses with similar genome structure and morphology [1]. In normal hosts, they cause a broad array of illnesses including conjunctivitis, upper and lower respiratory tract infection, pharyngitis with adenopathy, hemorrhagic cystitis, and occasionally meningoencephalitis. Although most of these infections occur in children, adults may also be affected. Epidemic, acute respiratory disease cause by serotypes 4 and 7 has been a significant problem among military trainees living in barracks. Recruits are now vaccinated with an effective live vaccine which is delivered orally in enteric-coated capsules.

Adenovirus was first isolated from the adenoids of a child in 1953 (hence its name). Latent or low-grade persistent infection may occur in lymphoid cells. Oncogenic transformation has also been described in vitro, but no role for adenoviruses in human tumorigenesis has been proven. Forty-one types of adenovirus have been described and these are segregated in six subgroups based on hemagglutination reactions. The most important immunity appears to be type-specific; accurate assessment of a patient's susceptibility to adenovirus infections involves testing for type by a neutralizing antibody assay. These viruses are important pathogens in immunocompromised hosts, particularly those with defective T-cell immunity. Adenovirus infections have been reported in solid organ and bone marrow transplant recipients but are not as common in these hosts as infections with herpes viruses such as cytomegalovirus. The severity of adenovirus infection can be very great, as demonstrated by the present case. The highest frequency of infection is seen in bone marrow recipients and pediatric liver transplant recipients. Table 24-1 shows the incidence of infection and disease due to adenoviruses in three large transplant studies (Refs. 2–4). The rate of infection was 5–10% in these populations, and fatal disease occurred in 1–2% of patients. By contrast, in adult solid organ transplant population the rate of infection is quite low.

The urinary tract is frequently involved in adenovirus infections. Clinically, one can see lower-tract involvement with hemorrhagic cystitis or upper-tract involvement with necrotizing nephritis. Serotypes 11 and 21 cause the majority of urinary tract infections. Why these types preferentially infect the urinary tract is unknown. Typical symptoms of hemorrhagic cystitis are gross hematuria, flank pain, and bladder spasms. Renal failure can ensue either because of obstruction from blood clots or direct involvement of the kidney. The presence of fever is often an indication of visceral involvement or dissemination to other organs. Our patient had a very large amount of virus in the urine (10^7) and had early clinical indication of disseminated disease in the lung and bowel.

In liver recipients, the most important complication of adenovirus infection is necrotizing hepatitis. Fever and moderate elevations of transaminases are generally present. Liver biopsy show well-circum-

Table 24-1. Adenovirus Infection and Disease in Selected Transplant Populations

Transplant Population	No. of Patients	Infected (% Tot)		Disease (% Tot)		Death (% Tot)	
Ped. liver	484	49	(10%)	20	(4%)	9	(2%)
Ped. liver	224	N/A		5	(2%)	2	(1%)
Bone marrow	1051	51	(4.9%)	10	(1%)	9	(1%)

Source: Adapted from Refs. 2–4.

scribed but scattered necrotic lesions with influx of acute and chronic inflammatory cells. Inclusion bodies may be seen and can be either eosinophilic or basophilic. A type of basophilic inclusion with shaggy borders called a "smudge cell" strongly suggests the diagnosis of adenovirus. Viral cultures of liver tissue and electron micrographs are other aids to a specific diagnosis. Other clinical syndromes caused by adenovirus are necrotizing enteritis and interstitial pneumonitis [5]. Mortality rates of greater than 50% are usually seen with adenovirus pneumonitis. Involvement of the lung is not easy to distinguish clinically from other causes of interstitial pneumonitis in transplant recipients, such as CMV infection. Also, most adenoviral infections occur between 1 to 4 months after transplantation at a time when cytomegalovirus (CMV) infection is also common. Some features that may differentiate adenovirus infection from CMV infection are the frequent involvement of the urinary tract and a greater severity of hepatitis in adenovirus infection.

In bone marrow recipients, graft-versus-host disease is thought to be an important risk factor for adenovirus disease. In solid organ recipients, adenovirus infections are much more common in pediatric populations, suggesting that acquired immunity in adults may provide a significant degree of protection. There is no approved treatment for adenovirus infection. The use of intravenous immunoglobulin may be tried and may be helpful if the patient is undergoing primary infection and has no endogenous circulating antibody against the virus. However, allogeneic marrow recipients, such as ours, have developed fatal adenovirus infection while receiving high doses of immunoglobulins. A few strains of adenovirus are susceptible to high levels of ganciclovir, in vitro. At this time, no clinical data support the use of ganciclovir [6]. Our patient continued to shed adenovirus while he was receiving ganciclovir. A decision to use ganciclovir must be balanced against the toxicity of the agent. Two novel antiviral compounds 2′-nor-cyclic GMP and (S)-9-(3-hydroxy-2-phosphonylmethoxypropyl) adenine [(S)-HPMPA] have excellent activity in vitro against a variety of adenovirus strains [7]. These agents have not undergone safety studies necessary to initiate clinical trials in humans. However, the demonstration of in vitro activity does indicate that effective antiviral therapy for adenovirus will likely be available in the future.

REFERENCES

1. Fox JP, Hall CE, Cooney MK. The Seattle Virus Watch. Observation of adenovirus infections. *Am J Epidem* 1977;105:362–386.

2. Shields AF, Hackman RC, Fife KH, Corey L, Meyers JD. Adenovirus infections in patients undergoing bone-marrow transplantation. *N Engl J Med* 1985;312:529–533.

3. Ambinder RF, Burns W, Forman M, Charache P, Arthur R, Beschorner W et al. Hemorrhagic cystitis associated with adenovirus infection in bone marrow transplantation. *Arch Intern Med* 1986;146:1400–1401.

4. Michael MG, Green M, Wald ER, Starzl TE. Adenovirus infection in pediatric liver transplant recipients. *J Infec Dis* 1992;165:170–174.

5. Zahradnik JM. Adenovirus pneumonia. *Semin Resp Infect* 1987;2:104–111.

6. Taylor DL, Jeffries DJ, Taylor-Robinson D, Parkin JM, Tyms AS. The susceptibility of adenovirus infection to the anti-cytomegalovirus drug, ganciclovir (DHPG). *FEMS Microbiol Lett* 1988;49:337–341.

7. Baba M, Mori S, Shigeta S, Clercq E. Selective inhibitory effect of (S)-9-(3-Hydroxy-2-phosphonylmethoxypropyl) Adenine and 2′-nor-cyclic GMP on adenovirus replication in vitro. *Antimicrob Agents Chemother* 1987;31:337–339.

25

Headache $1^1/_2$ Years After Bone Marrow Transplantation

Stephen Dummer and Steven Wolff

A 48-year-old man underwent allogeneic bone marrow transplantation for philadelphia chromosome positive chronic granulocytic leukemia in chronic phase. He received a marrow from his sister that was matched at five of six HLA loci. The conditioning regimen consisted of VP-16, cyclophosphamide, and total body irradiation. His initial posttransplant course was complicated by severe respiratory failure that was attributed to pulmonary toxicity from his chemotherapy. He required intubation for 4 days, but he eventually recovered and was discharged 51 days after transplantation. His medications at that time included cyclosporine 300 mg every 12 h and methylprednisolone 16 mg bid for graft-versus-host disease (GVHD) prophylaxis and sulfmethoxazole–trimethoprim (SMX-TMP) two double-strength tablets twice a week for prophylaxis against pneumocystis infection.

Two and one-half months after transplantation, the patient was admitted with fever, vomiting, and nausea that was exacerbated by movements of the head. A CT scan showed opacification of the mastoid air cells, most prominent on the right side, indicating mastoiditis. The patients symptoms resolved after treatment with oral antibiotics (ampicillin–clavulanate), antiemetic, and hydration. Five months later, the patient returned to the hospital with nausea, vomiting, and watery diarrhea of 2–3 weeks duration, and fever of 1 day duration. Sigmoidoscopy and upper endoscopy were performed. Biopsies of the stomach and rectum showed changes consistent with GVHD and he was treated with oral methylprednisolone 64 mg bid with improvement. In follow-up, the patient had intermittent symptoms of GVHD requiring continued treatment with oral corticosteroids.

One and one-half years after transplantation the patient was admitted to an outside hospital with a 4-week history of a continuous and worsening left parietal headache, associated with blurred vision and bilateral lower extremity weakness. Neurologic exam was normal except for slow mentation. A magnetic resonance scan of the brain showed a low density left temporal lobe lesion (Fig. 25-1). A lumbar puncture

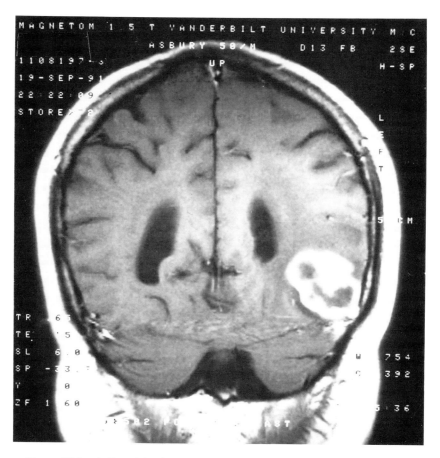

Figure 25-1.   A T$_1$-weighted magnetic resonance scan of the brain is shown in coronal orientation. A large multiloculated abscess is seen in the left temporal lobe.

yielded clear fluid with an opening pressure of 58 cm of water. The spinal fluid had one white blood cell, no red blood cells, a protein of 120 mg/dl, and glucose of 56. The patient was transferred to Vanderbilt University Medical Center. On physical exam here, his temperature was 97.8°F, pulse 88, respiration rate 20, and blood pressure 150/110. The remainder of the exam was remarkable for cushingoid facies and proximal lower extremity weakness. Admission medications included cyclosporine 240 mg orally, three times a week; methylprednisolone, 24 mg orally qod, SMX-TMP DS two tablets on Mondays and Thursdays, tenormin 50 mg/day, and ranitidine 150 mg bid.

LABORATORY EXAM

The results of the laboratory tests were as follows: sodium 138, potassium 4.1, bicarbonate 26, chloride 100, creatinine 1.0, BUN 27, white blood cell count 7000, with 88% neutrophils, hematocrit 35.0, and platelets 154,000. The chest radiograph showed normal heart size and no infiltrates. Review of the magnetic resonance scan (Fig. 25-1) showed a large abnormal signal, bright on T_2 and decreased on T_1 involving much of the left temporal lobe. There were three separate cavitary ring-like densities. A computerized tomographic scan of the brain showed strong ring enhancement of the lesion. Toxoplasma IgG titer was 1 : 32; toxoplasma IgM was negative.

HOSPITAL COURSE

The patient was started on broad-spectrum antibiotics designed to treat bacterial brain abscess, toxoplasmosis, and nocardiosis. The antibiotics included vancomycin 1 g, metronidazole 750 mg tid, ceftazidime 2 g tid, sulfadiazine 1 g qid, and pyrimethamine bid 100 mg loading dose and 25 mg a day thereafter. Three days later, he underwent stereotactic brain biopsy. The aspirate contained numerous neutrophils and branching gram-positive rods consistent with Nocardia species. The patients intravenous antibiotics were changed to Amikacin and cefotaxime. Oral sulfadiazine was continued. The nocardia isolate was sent the laboratory of Dr. Richard J. Wallace in Tyler, Texas who determined that it was *Nocardia nova*. Further in vitro testing at Dr. Wallace's laboratory showed it to be sensitive to amikacin, SMX-TMP, imipenem, sulfisoxazole, and ampicillin, intermediate in sensitivity to gentamicin, erythromycin, doxycycline, and cefotaxime, and resistant to ciprofloxacin, ampicillin–clavulanate, and minocyline. The patient's cefotaxime was discontinued, and he was placed on intravenous ceftriaxone 2 g q 12h. Over the next 2 weeks, the patients clinical status deteriorated slightly and he had intermittent episodes of somnolence. There was no change, however, in the appearance of brain CT scan. The sulfa level was 53 mg/dl. The sulfisoxazole dose was increased to 8 g a day, and the patient gradually improved. One month later, the amikacin was discontinued and the patient was discharged on the intravenous ceftriaxone and the oral sulfisoxazole. Three months after discharge, there was a marked decrease in the left temporal abscess. The intravenous ceftriaxone was discontinued, and the patient remained on oral sulfa medication while his corticosteroids were gradually tapered. Fourteen months after discharge, a CT scan of the brain showed no residual abscess, and daily sulfa therapy was discontinued.

DISCUSSION

This patient developed a space-occupying lesion of his left temporal lobe. The magnetic resonance and computerized tomographic scans were consistent with an abscess, although a necrotic tumor was another diagnostic possibility. The infections most likely to present in this fashion are routine bacterial brain abscess, nocardiosis, and aspergillosis. Toxoplasmosis was a less likely possibility. The patient's previous episode of mastoiditis made bacterial brain abscess a leading diagnosis at presentation. Otic infections are a known predisposing factor to bacterial brain abscess, especially in the temporal region of the brain. In cases like this, a rapid approach to a definitive diagnosis is crucial. A stereotactic aspiration yielded purulent material. A Gram stain of this material led to a definite diagnosis of nocardia infection and allowed initiation of therapy.

Nocardia is a soil bacterium that causes sporadic infection throughout the world. About half of the individuals who develop infection have some underlying condition affecting the immune system, and in most series, about 10–20% are transplant recipients. The largest series of nocardia infections in transplant recipients are in populations of renal and cardiac recipients. Cases in bone marrow recipients are only rarely described.

Nocardiosis is uncommon but not rare in renal recipients [1]. Most series describe the disease in 2–4% of transplant recipients. The incidence in a cohort of 160 heart recipients was much higher (13%) but dropped dramatically to 3% after cyclosporine was introduced in the early 1980s [2]. Many transplant physicians think the incidence of nocardia infection has fallen dramatically in recent years because of the widespread use of sulfa prophylaxis. It is, therefore, of interest that our patient was taking two double-strength tablets of sulfamethoxazole–trimethoprim twice a week when he presented with nocardiosis.

The portal of entry for nocardia is the lung [3]. Dissemination occurs in 20–25% of individuals. Pulmonary manifestations of infection are extremely variable and include bronchopulmonary infiltrates, nodules, which may be single or multiple, and cavitary lesions. Cavities are seen in about 20–25% of patients [4]. Pleural effusions, which may be sterile or infected, are present in 25–40% of patients with pulmonary nocardia infection. The most common site for dissemination is the central nervous system, and this is seen in about 15% of individuals with active infection. Single or multiple brain abscesses are the major manifestation. Meningitis may occur but is quite uncommon. The skin is the second most common site of dissemination and skin lesions usually present as mildly painful, palpable cold abscesses in the subcutaneous tissue.

Although bronchoscopy or open-lung biopsy may be required to make a diagnosis in some cases, the stain and culture of sputum are often adequate [5,6]. Growth of the organism usually takes 3–5 days but may take a number of weeks. Nocardia grows on most microbiological media, but because laboratories discard routine cultures by 48 h, it is wise to alert the microbiology laboratory to the possible presence of this organism.

The prognosis of nocardiosis is largely dependent on the presence or absence of central nervous system disease. In one large series, the mortality of nocardiosis with neurological involvement was 42%. Better results can be achieved when CNS dissemination is not present. At Stanford, none of 21 heart transplant patients with nocardia had central nervous system disease and none died directly of nocardia infection. Dissemination to subcutaneous tissue or other areas such as bone does not appear to confer a prognosis worse than isolated pulmonary disease.

The mainstay of therapy of nocardiosis is sulfa drugs [7]. There is little evidence that any oral sulfa drug is superior to any other, but sulfamethoxazole–trimethoprim is the preferred intravenous agent. Doses of sulfa from 4 to 8 g per day are used. Care should be taken to adjust doses for renal dysfunction. Sulfa levels are useful in patients with severe disease or renal dysfunction. We usually try to keep these in the range of 100 mcg/ml during the first few months of therapy. The optimum duration of treatment is not clear, but most authorities recommend prolonged therapy. We usually plan for 3–6 months of antibiotic therapy with isolated pulmonary disease and a year of therapy with central nervous system disease.

Many other antibiotics are active against nocardia. The decision to use additional agents depends on the overall status of the patient and the presence of dissemination. Amikacin is a drug that has very reliable activity against nocardia. Because of its toxicity, its use should probably be restricted to very severe cases. Other intravenous agents that are usually active are third-generation cephalosporins and imipenem. Minocycline is often cited as an alternative oral agent of choice, but experience with this drug in central nervous system disease is limited. If a patient has disseminated disease, it may be advisable to obtain antibiotic sensitivities on his isolate. This is best done at a reference laboratory, as most hospital laboratories have little experience performing sensitivities for this slow-growing organism.

The main caveats to be gleaned in this case are to always consider the disease when one or more lesions of the central nervous system are present because long-term cure can be achieved with aggressive diagnosis and therapy.

REFERENCES

1. Wilson JP, Turner HR, Kirschner KA, Chapman SW. Nocardial infections in renal transplant recipients. *Medicine* 1989;68:38–57.
2. Chapman SW, Wilson JP. Nocardiosis in transplant recipients. *Semin Resp Infect* 1990;5:74–79.
3. Petersen DL, Hudson LD, Sullivan K. Disseminated *Nocardia caviae* with positive blood cultures. *Arch Intern Med* 1978;138:1164–1165.
4. Simpson GL, Stinson EB, Egger MJ, Remington J. Nocardial infections in the immunocompromised host: A detailed study in a defined population. *Rev Infect Dis* 1981;3:492–507.
5. Palmer DL, Harvey RL, Wheeler JK. Diagnostic and therapeutic considerations in *Nocardia asteroides* infection. *Medicine* 1974;53:391–401.
6. Hall WA, Martinez AJ, Dummer JS, Lunsford DL. Nocardial brain abscess: Diagnostic and therapeutic use of stereotactic aspiration. *Surg Neurol* 1987;28:114–118.
7. Gombert ME. Susceptibility of *Nocardia asteroids* to various antibiotics, including newer beta-lactams, trimethoprim–sulfamethoxazole, amikacin, and N-formimidoyl thienamycin. *Antimicrob Agents Chemother* 1992;21:1011–1012.

Index